Safe Patient Handling and Movement

A Guide for Nurses and Other Health Care Providers

By Audrey L. Nelson, PhD, RN, FAAN

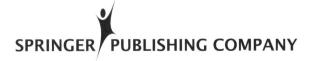

SPRINGER PUBLISHING COMPANY

This book is the result of work supported with resources and the use of facilities at the James A. Haley Veterans' Hospital, Tampa, Florida.

Springer Publishing Company, Inc.
11 West 42nd Street, 15th Floor
New York, NY 10036–8002

Acquisitions Editor: Ruth Chasek
Production Editor: Print Matters, Inc.
Composition: Compset, Inc.

07 08 09 10/5 4 3

Library of Congress Cataloging-in-Publication Data

Safe patient handling and movement : a guide for nurses and other health care
   providers / edited by Audrey L. Nelson.
        p. ; cm.
   Includes bibliographical references and index.
   ISBN 0-8261-6363-7
   1. Transport of sick and wounded.   2. Patients—Positioning.   3. Nursing.
      [DNLM: 1. Transportation of Patients—methods.   2. Accidents,
Occupational—prevention & control.   3. Back Injuries—prevention & control.
4. Safety Management—methods.   WY 100.2 S128 2006]
I. Nelson, Audrey, PhD.

RT87.T72S24 2006
610.73—dc22

2005056352

Printed in the United States of America by Bang Printing

Safe Patient Handling
and Movement

Contents

Part III: Special Challenges in Patient Handling

Part IV: Future Directions

Biosketches

James W. Collins, PhD, MSME, *Associate Director for Science*, 1095 Willowdale Road, Mail-stop 1900, Morgantown, WV 26505, is a Captain in the US Public Health Service and is the Associate Director for Science for the Division of Safety Research (DSR), with the Centers for Disease Control and Prevention (CDC), National Institute for Occupational Safety and Health (NIOSH). Dr Collins received his PhD in health policy and management from Johns Hopkins University and his masters and undergraduate degrees are in mechanical engineering. He has 21 years of experience as an engineer and an epidemiologist conducting laboratory and field research with the CDC/NIOSH. His recent research has focused on safe resident lifting in nursing homes and slip, trips, and falls prevention in hospitals.

William Charney, DOH, 5511 32nd Avenue NW, Apt. 102, Seattle, WA 98107, is currently the Safety Coordinator for Washington Hospital Services. He was the Director of Environmental Health for San Francisco General Hospital, Department of Public Health for the City and County of San Francisco. He has published six books on healthcare worker occupational health and safety, pioneered many new healthcare worker technologies used in the healthcare settings, and is the leading peer review author/researcher on lift teams.

Hans-Peter de Ruiter, RN, MS, Allina Hospitals and Clinics, MN, is Director of Nursing Research an Practice for the Allina Healthcare System and teaches nursing at a graduate and undergraduate level at the University of Minnesota and Excelsior College. Prior to this position he worked as Nurse Manager at the University of Minnesota Childrens Hospital and the Mayo Clinic. He was instrumental in developing and implementing a bariatric nursing care program at the Mayo Clinic. Hans-Peter has extensive direct patient care experience in pediactrics, acute medical care and mental health. From 2000 to 2001 he was program coordinator for a refugee mental health program in Thailand.

MaryAnn Burke de Ruiter, PT, MS, Courage Center, Golden Valley, MN, is employed at the Courage Center in Golden Valley, MN as a rehabilitation therapist. She has extensive experience in working with people with chronic conditions. MaryAnn has also worked with the Center of Victims of Torture in Minneapolis, and has supported torture victims by offering them physical therapy. In the period 1995–1998, she helped set up several physical therapy clinics in El Salvador.

Laureen G. Doloresco, MN, RN, CNAA-BC, *Associate Chief of Nursing for Spinal Cord Injury and Rehabilitation,* James A. Haley VA Hospital, 11605 N. Nebraska Avenue, Tampa, FL 33612, is Associate Chief of Nursing for Spinal Cord Injury and Rehabilitation Programs at the James A. Haley Veterans Hospital in Tampa, Florida, the first VA hospital to achieve national recognition by the American Nurses Credentialing Center (ANCC) for Magnet Nursing Services. Ms Doloresco has 29 years of nursing experience, including 19 years in nursing management and administration.

Guy Fragala, PhD, PE, CSP, *Director of Compliance Programs,* Environmental Health and Engineering, 60 Wells Avenue, Newton, MA 02459-3210, is currently Director of Compliance Programs with Environmental Health and Engineering in Newton, Massachusetts. He is retired from the faculty and his previous position as the Director of the Environmental Health and Safety Department at the University of Massachusetts Medical Center in Worcester, Massachusetts. He has consulted to a wide range of American industries and government agencies and authored numerous publications on the subjects of ergonomics and environmental health and safety. He has delivered many presentations on the subject of application of ergonomics to the healthcare industry. He has worked with the Patient Safety Center in Tampa, the Occupational Safety and Health Administration (OSHA), and the National Institute for Occupational Safety and Health (NIOSH) on safe patient handling issues. His book, *Ergonomics: How to Contain On-the-Job Injuries in Healthcare,* has been published and is being distributed by the Joint Commission on Accreditation of Healthcare Organizations.

John D. Lloyd, PhD, MErgS, CPE, *Associate Director,* Technology Innovations Division, VISN8 Patient Safety Center, James A. Haley Veterans' Hospital, Tampa, Florida serves as Director of the Research Laboratories and Associate Director of the Technology Division at the VISN8 Patient Safety Research Center in Tampa. John has served on multiple research projects, focusing on the prevention of musculoskeletal disorders through biomechanical evaluation and development of engineering solutions. He has recently been working on the development of a whole-body biomechanical model for analysis of dynamic human motion. This new technology has been utilized to describe the biomechanical stressors acting on upper extremity joints in persons with paraplegia during independent transfers.

Mary Matz, MSPH, IH, *VHA Patient Care Ergonomics Specialist*, VA Patient Safety Research Center, 11605 N. Nebraska Avenue (118M), Tampa, FL 33612-5738, is the Patient Care Ergonomic Program Specialist for the Veterans Health Administration (VHA). In this capacity, she provides patient care ergonomics consultation services and conducts training and ergonomic evaluations nationally, throughout VHA medical centers. She is an authorized OSHA instructor. She is a nationally recognized expert in patient care ergonomics and has co-authored several peer-reviewed papers on the subject. She received her BA in microbiology and MSPH in industrial hygiene from the University of South Florida.

Nancy N. Menzel, PhD, RN, *Assistant Professor*, Department of Healthcare Environments and Systems, College of Nursing, University of Florida, Box 100187, Gainesville, FL 32610, is an Assistant Professor of Community Health Nursing at the University of Florida College of Nursing. Her research focus is on psychosocial and behavioral interventions for musculoskeletal pain, injuries, and disability in direct patient care providers. She is a Certified Occupational Health Nursing Specialist, Certified Clinical Nurse Specialist in Community Health Nursing, and the author of two books on workers' compensation.

Jocelyn Villeneuve, BSc, Cert. SST, DESS, *Ergonomist*, ASSTSAS, 5100, rue Sherbrooke, Est, Bureau 950, Montreal (Quebec), Canada, H1V 3R9, is a senior ergonomist in a joint health and safety association in Montreal, Canada (ASSTSAS) where he leads an extensive program in ergonomics for healthcare facilities. He is a professor at Montreal University, where he graduated in health and safety. He also graduated from La Sorbonne University in Paris in ergonomics. He is past president of the Association of Canadian Ergonomists (ACE), Quebec, Canada.

Foreword

By Barbara Blakeney, MS, RN
President, American Nurses Association

As nurses, we often expect to make sacrifices for our careers and for our patients. While sacrificing our health should never be on that list, it is often a sad consequence of outdated teaching methods and ill-equipped facilities that do not offer devices known to protect staff from musculoskeletal disorders (MSDs). The problem is far from personal—in addition to affecting individual nurses, MSDs contribute to the nursing shortage and to insufficient patient care.

Research into the impact of MSDs on nurses has revealed that 52% of nurses surveyed complain of chronic back pain, while 12% say that they have left nursing "for good" because of back pain. Others who might join the nursing workforce are deterred by such daunting statistics. In a nation with a nursing shortage expected to increase to the point of 30% fewer nurses than needed by the year 2020, solutions must be put into action.

Fortunately, solutions do exist. The United States lags behind other nations in the use of safe lifting equipment. It is not just about keeping up with the international Joneses, though—it is about using existing equipment and technology to keep nurses and patients safe. And it is about educating policy makers, the workforce, and the nurses of tomorrow about safe patient handling. This is all within our grasp.

Assistive patient handling equipment may seem beyond the reach of many facilities struggling with their finances, but use of such equipment provides a benefit to all: the healthcare workers, their patients, and the healthcare facilities where they practice. Patients receive the benefits of reduced injuries, alleviated anxiety over awkward handling or positioning, and dignity left intact. Healthier nurses mean fewer absences, fewer nurses leaving the profession and, with luck, more men and women willing to join the profession.

This book addresses solutions to the problems posed by manual patient handling. It will define and outline the problem, offer general solutions, suggest methods of dealing with special needs patients, explore challenges related to particular healthcare settings, and offer tips for championing change. Use it not only to inform yourself and keep yourself safe, but also to start a dialogue about safe patient handling in your own facility or among your students. Use it to help your fellow nurses foresee a healthier future for themselves and their patients.

Preface

Since publication of the Institute of Medicine's (IOM) *To Err is Human: Building a Safer Health System* in 2000, the medical community, and the public at large has become more aware of issues surrounding patient safety. Yet there has been far less emphasis on caregiver safety. An estimated 12% of nurses leave the profession annually because of back injuries, and over half complain of chronic back pain. Yet there exists a panoply of techniques to reduce or eliminate this problem, the effectiveness of which has a solid research base, that can be currently implemented in patient care settings. These techniques include the use of technology, better architectural design of patient care space, and simple institutional policies (such as the use of lift teams). The reality is that patient safety cannot be fully addressed without considering caregiver safety. Consistent care is difficult to deliver with high turnover rates of staff, or increased rates of leave due to injuries, particularly at a time when there is a shortage of nurses.

This book was designed to present best practices in safe patient handling and movement, the current evidence base, and the scope of the problem. It also addresses the challenges of safe handling of special populations such as the morbidly obese. Nurse and hospital administrators, clinicians, clinical managers, risk managers, and those involved in the procurement and implementation of patient handling technologies into the healthcare environment will find this a practical resource for improving care and protecting staff from unnecessary injury.

In 2003, the American Nurses' Association (ANA) launched a "Handle with Care" ergonomics campaign to promote safe patient handling and the prevention of musculoskeletal disorders. In addition, since 2002, the Tampa Veterans Administration Hospital and the ANA have sponsored an annual Safe Patient Handling and Movement Conference. This book is an outgrowth of this effort within the nursing community to increase awareness of the serious problem of caregiver safety and available solutions.

I know that you will come away from reading this book with information that you can employ in a variety of work environments—hospitals, nursing homes, home care, and other health care organizations—whatever your practice setting may be. This is a resource guide that you can use as a training tool for new staff as well as a refresher for current staff. Opening these issues up for question and resolution in a patient care environment is an arduous but very rewarding task, and in the end, an essential exercise. Given the looming nursing shortage, implementation of these evidence-based strategies will be a crucial step in recruiting and retaining a competent nursing workforce.

Audrey L. Nelson, PhD, RN, FAAN

About the Editor

Audrey L. Nelson, PhD, RN, FAAN, *Director,* VA Patient Safety Research Center, 11605 N. Nebraska Avenue, Tampa, FL 33612-5738, has over 27 years of experience in nursing and currently serves as the Associate Chief of Nursing Service for Research at the Tampa VA, and Director of the Tampa Patient Safety Center of Inquiry. Dr Nelson is Associate Director of Clinical Research at the University of South Florida, College of Nursing, and is a Research Professor in the Colleges of Public Health and Engineering. She is a national leader in patient and caregiver safety. In 2005, Dr. Nelson was awarded the John Eisenberg Award for Patient Safety and Quality. Dr Nelson has expertise in research methods, safe patient handling and movement, wheelchair-related falls, and patient safety technology. She has had studies funded from the Veterans Health Administration, VA Health Services Research & Development and VA Rehabilitation Research and Development, OSHA, and Agency for Healthcare Research Quality (AHRQ).

Acknowledgment

I would like to acknowledge the stellar efforts of Valerie Kelleher, who assisted me in communications with authors, formatting early versions, and checking references cited throughout the book. She was instrumental in helping all of us to meet deadlines.

PART I

Introduction

Scope of the Problem

James W. Collins and Nancy N. Menzel

MOVING AND HANDLING PATIENTS: A CORE FUNCTION OF NURSES

In 1966, Virginia Henderson wrote a definition of nursing that clearly delineated the nursing profession from that of medicine:

> The unique function of the nurse is to assist the individual, sick or well, in the performance of those activities contributing to health or its recovery (or a peaceful death) that he would perform unaided if he had the necessary strength, will or knowledge. And to do this in such a way as to help him gain independence as rapidly as possible (p. 15).

During the course of most severe illnesses, afflicted individuals lose the ability to move on their own and require assistance for repositioning and movement. This responsibility falls to nursing care providers, who reposition patients to prevent pressure ulcers and promote comfort, put weakened limbs through range of motion to prevent contractures and promote circulation, ambulate patients to prevent blood clots and pneumonia, transfer patients to wheelchairs and stretchers so that they can travel to centralized services, and reposition bedridden patients as they bathe them, position patients for toileting, and reposition bedridden patients as linens are changed. Addressing patient mobility needs is a nursing function that can mean the difference between extensive complications or an uneventful recovery. Since the task of assisting patients with mobility deficits is inseparable from nursing care, it is essential to determine how nurses can perform these tasks safely.

A NEW APPROACH

A hundred years ago, this advice appeared in an early nursing textbook:

> "It is very good for strength
> To know that someone needs you to be strong."
> (Committee of the Connecticut Training-School for Nurses, 1906, preface verso).

In the 21st century, a new approach is recommended for patient handling and movement; it is not based on physical strength, but on the following principles:

1. The process of musculoskeletal pain, injury, and disability is affected by multiple causes involving the interaction of the caregiver, patient, and environment.
2. The lifting, transferring, and repositioning of patients can lead to fatigue, musculoskeletal pain, and disabling injuries.
3. The series of events involving the interaction of the patient, the caregiver, and the environment can be modified or interrupted to reduce the risk of injury to caregivers when lifting, transferring and repositioning patients.
4. Laboratory and field research have identified promising safe patient handling and movement (SPHM) programs that can greatly reduce the risk of injury to caregivers regardless of their age, length of employment, or shift.
5. SPHM programs can protect patients by reducing their risk of pain, skin tears, bruising, and being dropped.
6. A SPHM program is multi-faceted; it consists of mechanical equipment to lift and reposition patients, a safe-lifting policy, employee training on lift device usage, patient care assessment protocols and algorithms, unit-based peer safety leaders, and administrative support.
7. Periodic medical examinations should be performed on caregivers to identify musculoskeletal disorders early in their development.

These examinations should be conducted by healthcare providers who are knowledgeable about the caregiver's work exposures.

8. Administrative support and unit-based peer safety leaders are required to coordinate the resources and activities necessary for an effective SPHM program.

9. Although schools of nursing continue to teach manual patient handling methods, this new approach to patient handling and movement provides the information and tools necessary to support a paradigm shift in the nursing profession away from manual patient lifting and the over-reliance on body mechanics to multi-faceted SPHM programs.

HISTORY OF NURSING AND PATIENT HANDLING AND MOVEMENT

Since the emergence of professional nursing in Florence Nightingale's time, the musculoskeletal hazards of nursing work have not only been accepted as an inherent part of the job but also been blamed on the hapless (female) victim's lack of strength and poor lifting technique. In 1898, a standard nursing text exemplifies this mindset.

"Occasionally the complaint is made that a nurse has injured her back or strained herself in some way in moving a patient. This will generally be because she has failed to do the lifting properly" (Hampton, 1898, p. 102).

Amazingly, over 100 years later, "lifting properly," now known as body mechanics, is still the foundation of many of the educational programs for nursing students, despite the technological, scientific, and evidence-based revolution affecting all other aspects of care.

Although nurses have always been at risk for musculoskeletal injury, a significant rise in work-related disability can be traced to the shift in the nursing workplace from homes to hospitals and the change in how nursing care is delivered. Due to the reputation of hospitals as unclean facilities, only 10% of the sick were cared for in such institutions in 1915 (Joel & Kelly, 2002). Most nurses worked in private homes caring for a single patient. Long periods of bed rest were often the prescribed treatment, while patients were regarded as helpless, as is apparent from reading early nursing arts texts.

"Should a patient help himself? Not at all, if he is very ill. Never let him sit up or turn himself alone. Save his strength in every way" (Committee of the Connecticut Training-School for Nurses, 1906, p. 55).

With the advent of penicillin in the early 1940s, the reputation of hospitals began to change from one of high risk and last resort to a place of healing. More patients began receiving healthcare in hospitals rather than in their homes, resulting in a major post-World War II nursing shortage (Joel & Kelly, 2002). Due to the revolutionary concept of early ambulation, which made its way from the battlefield to hospitals sometime in the early 1940s (Sheldon & Blodgett, 1946), nurses found their workloads increasing from a single patient to a multitude of post-operative patients who had to be ambulated. Early ambulation increased the physical burden on nursing staff because they assisted unstable patients who could collapse or lose their balance with little notice. It was not long before articles about "aching backs" began to appear in nursing journals (Svec, 1951).

To meet the demand for bedside caregivers, hospitals reorganized nursing duties from the one-on-one model followed in the home by private duty nurses to a team concept. With the team concept, professional nurses had responsibility for a large number of patients, delegating some less-skilled tasks, such as ambulation and repositioning, to unlicensed assistive personnel. Exposure to lifting patients took its toll on these nursing aides and orderlies as well. Those with the job classification "nursing aides, orderlies, and attendants" are now reporting the highest number of musculoskeletal injuries with lost workdays in the US (US Bureau of Labor Statistics, 2004). Registered nurses (RNs) rank #7; it is the only professional group represented in the top 10 ranking.

The first citation in nursing for the phrase "body mechanics" appeared in the American Journal of Nursing in 1945 at the close of World War II. The author, a physician, wrote: "The recent appreciation of the value of reconditioning in the armed forces has stimulated a fresh interest in protective body mechanics for all patients" (Wright, 1945, p. 699). He added that "if nurses could be instructed in such a program," it could be "a protection to patients and themselves" (p. 703). Shortly thereafter, in 1946, a textbook appeared, *Body Mechanics in Nursing Arts*. This text contains many biomechanical illustrations of nurses shifting their weight while repositioning patients. The scientific foundation for this approach was absent. See Figure 1.1 for an example.

As the concept of body mechanics in nursing progressed, a 3-year demonstration project was published promoting "the value of the consistent use of good body mechanics to both nurses and patients" (Winters, 1950, p. 745). Winters (both an RN and a physical therapist) tried out a model curriculum at Vanderbilt University's School of Nursing and concluded that the 20-hour training program in body mechanics should be "an essential part of every nursing curriculum." Cited among the benefits to the student was learning to "use her own body efficiently

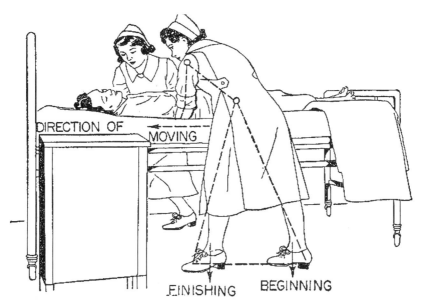

FIGURE 1.1 Illustration of body positioning in an early body mechanics text book (Fash, 1946).

to prevent unnecessary fatigue and strain" (Winters, 1950, p. 746). Like many traditions passed down through the legacy of nursing arts, there was no evidence presented that these techniques actually reduced fatigue and strain, let alone injury, or were safe for patients.

Lacking any evidence-based alternative to this approach to lifting and moving patients, yet facing the need to teach students how to handle and move patients, schools of nursing continued to emphasize body mechanics for the remainder of the 20th century and have continued teaching this approach into the 21st century. A 1958 practical nursing textbook stated: "Lifting does not always require strength. It takes skill which the nurse can readily develop once she has made good body mechanics a habit" (Gill, 1958, p. 299). Current fundamental nursing skills textbooks continue to include sections on body mechanics. Once the belief was established that proper body mechanics was a skill that would prevent musculoskeletal injuries, blaming the victim when an injury occurred was the logical inference.

Apparently the failure of proper body mechanics to protect nurses was due to more than lack of skill; it was also due to a physiological defect common among nurses. In 1965, a British researcher concluded that "the weak backs of nurses" were the reason injuries and sprains were so prevalent among the nursing profession ("Nurses have weak backs,"

1965). In contrast, in the same year, a British medical journal wrote an eloquent and enlightened editorial "The Nurse's Load" (1965, p. 422).

> The adult human form is an awkward burden to lift or carry. Weighing up to 100 kg or more, it has no handles, it is not rigid, and it is liable to severe damage if mishandled or dropped. In bed a patient is placed inconveniently for lifting, and the placing of a load in such a situation would be tolerated by few industrial workers. Since much of the nurse's day is spent in lifting patients, it is no small wonder that orthopedic wards often contain nurses with strained backs as patients.

Unfortunately, since Gill's work was published in the late 1950s, more than a million direct patient care providers have suffered from work-related back pain and disabling injuries. Even though the responsibility and blame for work-related injuries have fallen on the nursing profession, good body mechanics cannot always be used. For example, the "bent knees, straight back" method of lifting does not work well for lifting patients. When a patient is being lifted from a bed, the placement of the patient requires the caregiver to assume awkward postures and excessive forward bending. At the same time, the bed can restrict a nurse's ability to bend the knees. Other factors that can contribute to the difficulty of lifting a patient are the size and weight of the patient, the patient's propensity to fall or lose balance, the bed height, patient combativeness and/or their inability to help. Additionally, the vast majority (90%) of the lifting and moving of physically dependent patients is performed by female nursing staff (Lloyd, 2004; US Department of Labor, 2004) who lack the upper body strength of men.

CONSEQUENCES OF MUSCULOSKELETAL INJURIES IN NURSING PERSONNEL

Nurses are clearly concerned about becoming injured during the performance of their work. The basis for their fear is that a back injury can end their careers and earning capacity (Helminger, 1997). In a 2001 study conducted by the American Nurses Association, 4826 nurses cited "disabling back injury" as their second highest health and safety concern; "stress and overwork" was listed as number one. Consequences to employers include the high costs of workers' compensation insurance to pay for medical care and days away from work for injured workers, as well as the need to hire replacement workers (Menzel, 1998). Protecting the health and safety of nursing personnel is vital not only to the staff members and their employers but also to the nation's health. An insufficient number of hospital nursing staff, a problem that is exacerbated by loss of nursing staff due to back injuries, results in an increased risk of deaths and complications among hospitalized patients (Aiken, Clarke, Sloane, Sochalski, & Silber, 2002; Needleman, Buerhaus, Mattke, Stewart, & Zelevinsky, 2002).

THE EXTENT OF MUSCULOSKELETAL PROBLEMS IN NURSING PERSONNEL

In 1985, Harber and associates surveyed over 500 nurses in a California hospital and found that over half had experienced back pain in the previous 3 months. A random sample of licensed nurses in Wisconsin by Owen (1989) found that 52% of hospital nurses experienced work-related low-back pain in the past year; 48% of these stated that lifting and repositioning patients in bed had precipitated their low-back pain. In 2001, a survey of 113 direct patient care providers in a Florida Veterans Health Administration (VHA) facility found current musculoskeletal discomfort of at least moderate severity in 62% of the direct patient care staff (Menzel, Brooks, Bernard, & Nelson, 2004). In 2002, a survey of over 1100 RNs found that 47% experienced back pain in the previous year (Trinkoff, Lipscomb, Geiger-Brown, & Brady, 2002).

The musculoskeletal injury problem among nurses is not unique to the United States. Epidemiological studies around the world have consistently identified nursing personnel at high risk of low-back pain and musculoskeletal injury (Menzel, 2004). In England, Stubbs, Buckle, Hudson, Rivers, & Worringham (1983) reported that 43% of nursing personnel suffer from low-back pain annually, twice as much as the general population, and attributed 84% of these episodes to moving or supporting a patient. It is estimated that 16% of the sick leave taken by nurses in England is due to back pain (Pheasant & Stubbs, 1992). One study showed that 18% of nursing personnel stopped working because of low-back pain (Videman et al., 1984). A study of 3159 young (mean age 24.8) nurses in Taiwan found the 1-year prevalence of back pain to be 69.7% (Lee & Chiou, 1994). In Greece, researchers found a 1-year prevalence of back pain of 75% in that country's nurses (Alexopoulos, Burdorf, & Kalokerinou, 2003).

Even though the rates of injury reported by caregivers in hospitals and nursing homes are excessively high, it is suspected that there is significant underreporting. Many nurses work with musculoskeletal pain but do not file claims. Cato, Olson, and Studer (1989) found that 78% of nurses with back pain in the previous 6 months did not report it to management, while Owen (1989) found that 67% (126 of 189) of nurses suffering from low-back pain related to work did not report the incident in writing

(Owen, 1989). Student nurses have reported back pain related to "heavy" work on patient units (Klaber-Moffett, Hughes, & Griffiths, 1993).

THE RISKS OF WORKING AT HOSPITALS AND NURSING HOMES

Since 1980, the Bureau of Labor Statistics (BLS) has recorded injury and illness rates in hospitals and nursing homes (Personick, 1990). In the 1980s, the nursing home and personal care industry consistently incurred more than 100,000 non-fatal occupational injuries and illnesses. The epidemic of injuries in nursing and personal care facilities led the BLS to commission a series of studies in 1988 focusing on industries with the largest numbers of workplace injuries and illnesses (Personick, 1990). The first of these studies was initiated in the Nursing and personal care industry due to the high number of injuries and because 1988 marked the sixth consecutive annual increase in injury rates in nursing homes. As shown in Figure 1.2, from 1980 to 1992, the injury incidence rate for hospitals and nursing homes steadily increased and has steadily declined since the mid 1990s. Personick noted that incidence rates steadily increased from 10.7 per 100 workers in 1980 to a peak of 18.6 per 100 workers in 1992 (US Department of Labor, 1994).

**Injuries per 100 full-time workers
in hospitals and nursing and personal care facilities
1980-2002**

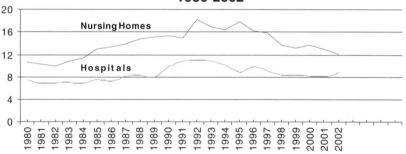

SOURCE: U.S. Department of Labor, Bureau of Labor Statistics.

FIGURE 1.2 Injuries per 100 full-time workers in hospitals and personal care facilities (Source: U.S. Department of Labor, Bureau of Labor Statistics)

The risk of back pain has been consistently higher in nursing homes than hospitals, presumably because residents require more physical assistance from nursing staff members to perform their activities of daily living, such as getting in and out of beds or chairs, bathing, and toileting. In addition, there are usually fewer staff members per number of patients in nursing homes versus hospitals, increasing the lifting exposure for individual workers. The majority of the industry's reported injuries were serious enough to require time off from work or restrict a caregiver's work activity. Of the 151,000 injuries and illnesses reported in nursing homes in 1988, approximately 88,000 resulted in lost work time (Personick, 1990). The tenure of the injured worker in the nursing home tended to be relatively short (less than 1 year) at the time of the incident (Personick, 1990; Collins, Wolf, Bell, & Evanoff, 2004). The highest injury rates in nursing homes occurred among nursing assistants less than 25 years old.

It is not clear what contributed to the steady increase in injury rates prior to 1992; however, in the early to mid 1990s research efforts increasingly began to focus on the prevention of musculoskeletal injuries among healthcare workers. The steady increase in musculoskeletal injuries prompted nursing homes and hospitals to examine ways to contain the escalating workers' compensation costs. Around this same time, the Occupational Safety and Health Administration began to target nursing and personal care facilities as part of a special emphasis program citing imminent hazards due to patient lifting under the "general duty clause." In response to a perceived demand for better equipment to lift and transfer patients, healthcare equipment manufacturers responded by improving existing patient lifting equipment and by developing an extensive amount of new patient handling technology.

Although no studies have formally examined factors affecting the trends in nursing home and hospital injury rates since 1980, it is suspected that a number of factors have affected the fluctuations in injury rates. During the late 1980s, the issue of musculoskeletal injuries in nursing homes was drawing international attention. The National Institute for Occupational Safety and Health (NIOSH) began to sponsor feasibility studies on how to reduce musculoskeletal injuries related to patient handling in healthcare settings (Garg & Owen, 1992). Since 1993, the incidence rate in nursing homes has steadily declined with consecutive decreases in all but one of the past 10 years (Figure 1.2).

The results of an Institute of Medicine study (1986), *Improving the Quality of Care in Nursing Homes*, directly led to the nursing home reform provisions in the Omnibus Budget Reconciliation Act of 1987. The law was enacted to upgrade the staff requirements for US nursing homes certified by Medicare or Medicaid. The law mandated that, by 1990, nursing homes must provide licensed nursing services during all hours and that nursing aides must complete at least 75-hours of training in nursing skills and residents' rights. The result was the most far-reaching revision to the standards, inspection process, and enforcement system since the passage of Medicare and Medicaid in the mid 1960s (Hawes, 1990). The new standards spoke to the process of care that was expected and to the requirement that care would promote "the maximum practicable functioning" for each individual resident. Federally mandated staffing standards may have prompted nursing homes to increase staff retention by improving working conditions by providing more mechanical lifting equipment.

In addition to these regulatory forces, increases in workers' compensation costs forced hospitals and nursing homes to consider ways to return injured employees to work in modified duty status, thereby avoiding paying indemnity (wage replacement) (Menzel, 1998). Because the BLS tracks injuries involving days away from work, it is likely that this movement toward modified duty has reduced the number of injured workers recorded as missing time from work. The following sections discuss what is causing these injuries.

Occupational Risk Factors

An assessment of workers' compensation claims for back strains and sprains concluded that nursing aides and practical nurses ranked in the 10 occupations with the highest rate of back strains or sprains claims. Only heavy laborers, such as garbage collectors and warehouse workers, ranked higher than nursing personnel (Klein, Jensen, & Sanderson, 1984). Within categories of direct patient care providers, certified nursing aides (CNAs) and orderlies suffered the highest rates of musculoskeletal injury followed by licensed practical nurses (LPNs) and then RNs (Jensen, 1987). When examining injury rates for female workers in the United States, nursing aides and orderlies have the highest prevalence (18.8%) and report most cases of work-related back pain of all occupations (Guo et al., 1995). In contrast to services provided by hospitals, the nature of patient care in nursing homes calls for substantially more nursing aides than LPNs or RNs. The high risk of back pain among CNAs, can be attributed to job-related exposure to high-risk tasks; their job includes provision of "basic care and duties such as feeding, bathing, dressing, grooming, or moving patients under the direction of nursing staff" (US Department of Labor, 2002). In contrast, the job descriptions for RNs and LPNs include assessing patient health problems and providing nursing care to the ill, but make no mention of moving patients (US Department of Labor, 2004). Contrary to this inexplicable omission in BLS's occupational classification, many RNs and LPNs perform patient handling and movement tasks as part of their regular responsibilities.

The increase in nursing workloads has continued to the present. With higher levels of patient acuity and shorter hospital stays, today's hospitalized patients are more dependent on nurses to assist them with mobility needs. Due to the pronounced trend of discharging the less seriously ill to recuperate elsewhere, the average length of hospital stay declined from 7.5 days in 1980 to 4.9 days in 2001, concentrating the number of sick people who need more assistance in acute care facilities (National Center for Health Statistics, 2003). Yet there have been few innovations in nursing practice or hospital infrastructure since World War II to assist direct patient care staff in caring for this increasingly dependent patient population.

Personal Risk Factors for Musculoskeletal Injury and Low-Back Pain in Nurses

When musculoskeletal injuries in nursing personnel are examined by occupation, age, gender, length of employment, and other potential risk factors, certain subgroups of nursing personnel emerge at higher risk for sustaining injury. A study of work-related injury in the Central Arkansas Veterans Healthcare System examined medical center employee injuries from 1998 to 2000 in terms of age, gender, employment type, employment status, shift length, body mass index (BMI), workers' compensation claims prior to current employment, employee health and wellness activity attendance, lost time claims, and medical/loss of productivity costs (Brown & Thomas, 2003). Notable characteristics of injured employees included advancing age, female gender, long working hours, increased BMI, history of prior back and upper extremity injuries, no health and wellness activity attendance, and lost time with injury. Back and shoulder strain, falling-related injuries, and repetitive motion injuries were the most severe and costly injuries. The association between BMI and musculoskeletal injuries in nursing personnel has not been seen by other researchers (Smedley, Egger, Cooper, & Coggon, 1997).

Authors of one study examined a range of etiologic risk factors, including personal and work-related factors, and identified heavy lifting, work experience, age, work knowledge, work habits, and sitting habits to be significant predictors of back pain. Heavy lifting was found to be the most significant risk factor for nursing back pain (Lee & Chiou, 1994). Specifically, the results showed that the more and heavier the patients lifted, the older the nurse, the longer the work experience, the poorer the knowledge of work postures, the poorer the work habits, and the poorer the sitting habits, the higher the 1-year prevalence of low-back pain. Venning et al. (1987) examined the contribution of personal and job-related factors as determinants of back injuries in 5469 nurses. Factors found to be significant predictors of back injury included greater exposure to frequent lifting, working as a nursing aide versus an RN, and a previous history of back injury, suggesting that job-related factors rather than personal factors are the major predictors of back injury in nurses.

When examining 416 back injury reports at an 1100-bed acute and tertiary care hospital, the rate of injury among 1645 nurses was found to be highest for those working on orthopedic, medicine, neurology, spinal, and surgery wards (Yassi et al., 1995). In fact, 51% of the orthopedic nurses sustained at least one back injury during the 2-year study period. Gender did not significantly affect the risk of back injury; however, injuries were slightly more common in nurses with less seniority, and younger nurses were at a significantly increased risk of back injury. Lifting and transferring patients with assistance were the two most common activities for back injury (22.6% and 23.3%, respectively). Injured nurses attributed 52.3% of their injuries to inadequate training; inadequate staffing was given as the primary reason for 13.8% of the injuries. In a large-teaching hospital, the total injury rate for nurses ranged from 14.2 per 100 nurses in the intensive care unit to 3.8 per 100 nurses in the pediatric unit (Goldman, Jarrard, Kim, Loomis, & Atkins, 2000).

Environmental and Physical Risk Factors

In addition to the heavy lifting and physical demands associated with manually lifting patients, the forward bending, twisting, and reaching required when feeding, bathing, and dressing patients are also associated with an increased risk of musculoskeletal injury (Harber et al., 1987; Owen & Garg, 1991). The height of the bed has an important influence on the working posture and handling capacity of nurses (Lee & Chiou, 1994). Simple nursing tasks such as measuring blood pressure and giving injections at the bedside can generate high static loads on the musculoskeletal system of nurses (Harber et al., 1987).

Lifting and moving patients manually has been identified as a high-risk activity (Agnew, 1987; Garg, Owen, & Carlson, 1992; Marras, Davis, Kirking, & Bertsche, 1999; Nelson & Fragala, 2004; Zhuang, Stobbe, Hsiao, Collins, & Hobbs 1999; Stubbs, Rivers, Hudson, & Worringham, 1981). Moving or lifting a patient in bed was perceived to have precipitated 61% of the low-back pain episodes and 60% of the lost workdays (Owen, 1989).

Changes in Work Organization

The healthcare industry has undergone sweeping organizational changes. The increase in managed care has resulted in shorter hospital stays and sicker hospitalized patients with higher levels of acuity. Between 1981 and 1993, total hospital employment grew steadily, whereas the number of nursing personnel employed declined by 7.3% (Lipscomb, Trinkoff, Brady, & Geiger-Brown, 2004). In a cross-sectional study of 1163 nurses, it was found that nurses who reported that the healthcare system where they worked underwent more than six organizational changes also reported significantly more musculoskeletal disorders involving the neck, back, and shoulders when compared to nursing staff who reported no more than one change in the way their work was organized (Lipscomb et al., 2004). The Minnesota Nurses Association found that when RN positions in hospitals decreased by 9%, the number of work-related injuries or illnesses among RNs in those hospitals increased by 65% (Shogren, Calkins, & Wilburn, 1996).

Evolution of Prevention Effectiveness Research

Ineffectiveness of Body Mechanics Training. Training alone has not been shown to reduce the risk of patient-lifting related injuries to nursing personnel (Dehlin & Lindberg, 1976; Dehlin, Berg, Anderson, & Grimby, 1981; Nelson, Fragala, & Menzel, 2003a; Snook, Campanelli, & Hart, 1978; Wood, 1986). Research on healthcare worker back injuries has progressed from the early work that described the injury prevalence and incidence by job title, age, gender, and other demographic characteristics (Cust, Pearson, & Mair, 1972) to examining the effectiveness of training programs. After it became widely recognized that the hazard of lifting heavy human bodies could not be alleviated by training alone, subsequent studies examined patient lifting from an ergonomic viewpoint; researchers began conducting task analyses and biomechanical evaluations of patient handling activities with the intent of redesigning and adapting patient handling tasks to not exceed the capacities of caregivers.

Task Analyses. Task analyses are one of the tools used to conduct ergonomic assessments to evaluate methods used for lifting and transferring patients. From the perspective of epidemiology, task analyses provide an assessment of the caregiver's exposure to physical risk factors that can contribute to musculoskeletal disorders. The capacity of a caregiver to perform the requirements of lifting tasks requires an understanding of the biomechanical forces, postures, the hand grip a nurse holds a patient with, the vertical height a patient is lifted and the distance a patient is moved (Waters, Putz-Anderson, Garg, & Fine, 1993).

For patient handling, aspects of the lifting task that must be considered include the weight of the patient, the weight-bearing ability of the patient, and the posture and the type of grip that the caregiver has on the patient while lifting. The challenge of lifting and moving patients is further complicated by the patient's size, shape, level of fatigue, cognitive functioning, cooperation as well as the worker's physical impairments, lower limb function, balance, and coordination (Lloyd, 2004). Cognitively impaired patients can be unpredictable. They may abruptly struggle or resist the caregiver, or become limp during a transfer, creating a sudden unexpected load on the caregiver (Lloyd, 2004). This sudden loading can cause excessively high forces that can injure the spinal muscles (Anderson 2001). Task analyses conducted in nursing homes identified the most physically demanding tasks as transferring physically dependent residents to and from the toilet, in and out of beds and chairs, repositioning in bed, and transfers for bathing and weighing residents (Garg et al., 1992).

Biomechanical Laboratory Studies.   Historically, the caregiver has used his or her own physical strength to provide manual assistance to the patient. In 1987, Bell indicated that patient lifts had been available for 100 years, but it was not until the early 1990s that published studies began to demonstrate that the risk of injury to caregivers in nursing homes could be reduced through the use of mechanical lifting equipment.

Extensive research has documented high levels of biomechanical stress on caregivers when performing patient lifting and repositioning tasks (Gagnon, Sicard, & Sirois, 1986; Lloyd, 2004; Marras et al., 1999; Ulin et al., 1997; Zhuang et al., 1999). A biomechanical evaluation of nine battery-powered lifts, two assistive devices, and a manual baseline method for transferring nursing home residents from a bed to a chair revealed that the method of transfer and the resident's weight affected a nursing assistant's low-back loading (Zhuang et al., 1999). The use of portable or ceiling-mounted mechanical lifts significantly reduced the nursing assistants' back compressive forces and removed about two-thirds of the exposure to lifting activities per transfer as compared to the baseline manual method (Zhuang et al., 1999).

Laboratory-based biomechanical studies have identified safer ways to lift and move patients by removing the excessive forces and extreme postures that can occur when manually lifting patients. The collective assessment of the biomechanical laboratory studies led to the conclusion that mechanical lifting equipment could significantly reduce the biomechanical stress that lead to musculoskeletal injuries when compared to manual methods (Garg et al., 1992; Harber et al., 1985; Marras et al., 1999; Owen, 1987; Zhuang et al., 1999).

Field Studies and Demonstration Projects. The research literature on back and musculoskeletal injuries among nurses has been expanding rapidly since the 1980s. More recently, the emphasis on nursing back injury research has shifted from describing the magnitude of the problem to seeking solutions to eliminate the problem. After laboratory studies demonstrated that mechanical lifting equipment could significantly reduce the physical stresses imposed on caregivers under controlled conditions in the laboratory, the next phase of research was to validate the effectiveness of mechanical lifting equipment in real-world settings. The most recently published studies have been field studies conducted in hospitals and nursing homes. A strong body of intervention effectiveness research has been amassed demonstrating that mechanical lifting equipment as part of a SPHM program can significantly reduce musculoskeletal injuries among healthcare workers (Collins et al., 2004; Garg, 1999; Garg & Owen, 1992; Nelson & Fragala, 2004; Yassi et al., 2001).

One of the first comprehensive intervention evaluation studies demonstrating the effectiveness of mechanical lifting equipment in the context of a comprehensive program was funded by the NIOSH and conducted by Garg & Owen, (1992). The program evaluation included:

- Identifying the most stressful patient handling tasks
- Performing an ergonomic evaluation of these tasks
- Conducting a laboratory study to select less stressful patient transferring tasks
- Conducting a field study to evaluate mechanical lifting equipment
- Training nursing staff how to use the equipment
- Modifying toilets and shower rooms
- Applying the techniques to resident care

The authors concluded that ergonomic intervention programs were effective in reducing the risk of low-back pain in the small sample of nursing personnel in the study, and stated that large-scale studies in different nursing homes were needed to confirm the above findings. Building on these findings, a larger study assessed the long-term effectiveness of patient handling programs in seven nursing homes and one hospital (Garg, 1999). Fifty-one months after the resident lifting program was introduced, injuries from resident transfers decreased by 62%, lost workdays by 86%, restricted workdays by 64%, and workers' compensation costs by 84%.

In a study conducted by the NIOSH (Collins et al., 2004), a safe resident handling and movement program reduced resident-handling workers' compensation injury rates by 61%, lost workday injury rates by 66%, and restricted workdays by 38%. Additionally, the number of workers suffering from repeat injuries was reduced. During the 36 months before the intervention there were 129 workers' compensation claims attributed to resident handling, and 11 workers filed more than one workers' compensation claim for musculoskeletal injuries. During the 36-month post-intervention period, 56 workers' compensation claims were attributed to resident handling and only 3 employees filed more than one workers' compensation claim associated with resident handling tasks.

The VHA conducted an evaluation of ceiling-mounted patient lifts on a 60-bed nursing home unit deemed to be "high risk" based on the number and severity of injuries reported over a 2-year period (Tiesman, Nelson, Charney, Siddharthan, & Fragala, 2003). At 18-months post-intervention, the incidence of injuries was slightly lower; however, lost workdays were reduced to zero. Subjective ratings by caregivers indicated a high level of satisfaction with the program.

In a separate study, (Nelson et al., 2003b), a multi-faceted program was evaluated in 23 high-risk long-term care units in seven VHA facilities with 780 nursing personnel. The multi-faceted program included mechanical patient lifts, patient care assessment protocols, no-lift policies, and training on the proper use of patient handling equipment. During the post-intervention period, there was a significant decrease in the rate of injuries and modified duty days, an increase in caregiver satisfaction, and a decrease in the number of "unsafe" patient handling practices performed daily, as reported by nurses. Ninety-six percent of the nurses ranked lifting equipment as the most important program element.

A randomized controlled trial compared the effectiveness of training and equipment to reduce musculoskeletal injuries, increase comfort, and reduce physical demands on staff performing patient lifts and transfers at a large acute care hospital (Yassi et al., 2001). This randomized controlled trial consisted of a "control" group, a "safe lifting" group, and a "no strenuous lifting" group. Both intervention groups received intensive training in back care, patient assessment, and handling techniques, whereas the no strenuous lifting group added mechanical lifts and other assistive equipment. The frequency of manual patient handling tasks was significantly decreased in the no strenuous lifting group. Self-perceived work fatigue, back and shoulder pain, safety, and frequency and intensity of physical discomfort associated with patient handling tasks were improved on both intervention groups, but staff in the no strenuous lifting group showed greater improvements.

A study was conducted in the extended care unit of a hospital to examine the marginal benefit of replacing a traditional floor lift patient lifting program with overhead ceiling lifts (Ronald et al., 2002). During the pre-intervention period there were five mechanical floor lifts, one manual transfer aid, and four beds serviced by two ceiling lifts. After completion of the resident lifting program, the unit included 3 floor lifts, 62 ceiling lifts, and 3 tubs serviced by ceiling lifts. The rate of musculoskeletal injuries caused by lifting/transferring patients was significantly reduced by 58% after the installation of ceiling-mounted lifts, but the rate of musculoskeletal injuries caused by repositioning did not decline. Although the ceiling lifts are designed for both lifting and repositioning residents, the ceiling lifts were actually not used for repositioning residents because of problems with the repositioning slings. Neither equipment nor environmental factors represented major causal factors for musculoskeletal injury pre- or post-intervention. Resistive behavior by patients was the major patient-related causal factor.

CASE MANAGEMENT OF INJURED WORKERS

One of the early field studies in Canada evaluated the effectiveness of a "Personnel Program" that was designed as a case management program to increase communication between injured workers, their doctors, the workers' compensation board, and the hospital administration (Wood, 1986). The Personnel Program significantly reduced the proportion of claims resulting in more than 1000 hours away from work (7.1% to 1.7%) and the frequency of claims filed for incidents. The author attributed the success of the program to carefully documenting and coordinating the complex interactions between the injured worker, the workers' compensation board, the doctors, and the hospital. The program also made a clear statement to workers: "As an employee of this hospital, you are our most valued resource and we cannot afford to replace you."

The findings of a study of 416 nursing back injuries at a large-teaching hospital in Canada add to the evidence that a return to work program can be effective in reducing the duration of time loss due to work-related back injuries (Tate, Yassi, & Cooper, 1999).

DEMONSTRATING COST–BENEFIT
OF SPHM PROGRAMS

The establishment of safe patient lifting and movement programs not only provides benefits to caregivers and patients, but also makes good business sense. Cost–benefit analyses from study data demonstrate that the initial investment in lifting equipment and employee training can be recovered in 2–4 years through reductions in workers' compensation expenses. In a study in six nursing homes, the total capital investment in equipment was $143,556 and an estimated $15,000 was invested in training employees on how to use the equipment (Collins et al., 2004). Each nursing home spent an average of $26,500 on lifting equipment and employee training. The average annual savings in workers' compensation costs due to a reduction in employee injuries related to resident handling was $9150. Because the healthcare system was self-insured, the reduction in workers' compensation expenses was recovered immediately, rather than as a reduction in insurance premiums in future years. The reduction in workers' compensation expenses recovered the initial capital investment in slightly less than 3 years. The return on investment is even shorter if savings in indirect costs are considered (e.g., lost wages, cost of hiring and retraining workers).

An evaluation of a SPHM program among 780 nursing personnel from 23 high-risk long-term care units in 7 VHA facilities showed that equipment and training costs were recovered in saved workers' compensation expenses in approximately 24 months (Nelson et al., 2003b; Tiesman et al., 2003). In a study that evaluated resident lifting programs in seven nursing homes and one hospital (Garg, 1999), the sharp decrease in workers' compensation costs resulted in an average payback period of 15 months (range 5–29 months).

The impact of installing 65 ceiling-mounted lifts was evaluated in the extended care unit of a hospital in British Columbia; the aim was to determine if musculoskeletal injuries were reduced among healthcare workers (Spiegel et al., 2002). The ceiling-mounted lifts were purchased with a one-time capital expenditure of $344,323. Workers' compensation costs associated with lifting and transferring residents were reduced by 69% or $89,378 annually, resulting in a payback period of 3.85 years. Spiegel noted that whereas financial analyses are useful, they should not be the only factor in making program decisions. Qualitative information related to the well-being of the workforce and residents should be considered as well. The economic information generated by this study did not serve as the sole decision-making criterion, but rather was used in conjunction with qualitative nursing and patient issues. Installation of overhead mechanical lifting equipment is currently being considered as a possible standard for newly constructed hospitals in Canada.

INACTION AND INJURY

Despite the evidence of the effectiveness of these interventions, hospitals have been slower than nursing homes to adopt such programs, often citing the financial cost of equipment and associated training. Schools of nursing continue to teach manual handling methods, and many hospitals do not have mechanical aides to assist with patient transfers. Nursing licensure examinations continue to test nursing school graduates on manual handling, as is indicated by this statement from the 2004 NCLEX-RN Test Plan: "Use correct body mechanics to lift, transfer, transport, position and assist clients to ambulate" (National Council of State Boards of Nursing, 2003). Employers in the healthcare industry should work together to reduce the lifting burden for their employees. Likewise, educators should teach patient handling techniques based on the research evidence demonstrating the effectiveness of SPHM programs. State boards of nursing should discontinue testing prospective licensees on manual lifting methods that have been proven to be ineffective. With hospital nursing vacancies projected to be 800,000 by 2020 (Health Resources and Services Administration, 2002), nurses are a valuable resource that should be protected through the widespread implementation of SPHM programs.

SUMMARY

Since most schools of nursing continue to teach manual patient handling methods, and nurses tend to practice what they were taught in school, a paradigm shift is necessary to change the way patients are lifted and transferred. Because nursing homes and hospitals are beginning to implement ergonomics programs on a widespread basis in the United States, some nursing personnel have modified their patient lifting work practices. With the collaborative assistance of the nursing licensure boards and schools of nursing, this book can be a stimulus for changing the way patient lifting and the biomechanics of lifting patients are taught to nursing students.

Although musculoskeletal injury rates to nursing personnel vary by age, gender, length of employment, and job title, prevention strategies should provide protection for all nursing personnel regardless of age, height, or other pre-disposing factors. A body of research has been accumulating that supports a multi-faceted approach to reducing the risk of patient handling injuries to caregivers. Teaching professionals need to replace manual patient handling methods taught in outdated biomechanical classes with the SPHM principles presented in the following chapters. These principles include ergonomic assessments of patient handling activities, patient assessment and use of algorithms, redesigning patient lifting tasks by utilizing new patient handling technology, use of unit-based peer safety leaders, and administrative support in the context of a SPHM program. With a SPHM program, nursing care providers can enjoy the rewards of their work free from pain and injury.

REFERENCES

Agnew, J. (1987). Back pain in hospital workers. In E. Emmett (Ed.), Health problems of health care workers. *Occupational Medicine State of the Art Reviews, 2*(3), 609–616.

Aiken, L. H., Clarke, S. P., Sloane, D. M., Sochalski, J., & Silber, J. H. (2002). Hospital nurse staffing and patient mortality, nurse burnout, and job dissatisfaction. *JAMA, 288*, 1987–1993.

Alexopoulos, E. C., Burdorf, A., & Kalokerinou, A. (2003). Risk factors for musculoskeletal disorders among nursing personnel in Greek hospitals. *International Archives of Occupational and Environmental Health, 76*(4), 289–294.

American Nurses Association. (2001). Nurses cite stress, overwork as top health, safety concern. *The American Nurse, 33*, 1, 8.

Anderson, B. T. (2001). Sudden movements of the spinal column during health-care work. *International Journal of Industrial Ergonomics, 28*(1), 47–53.

Bell, F. (1987). Ergonomic aspects of equipment. *International Journal of Nursing Studies, 24*(4), 331–337.

Brown, N. D., & Thomas, N. I. (2003). Exploring variables among medical center employees with injuries: developing interventions and strategies. *AAOHN Journal, 51*(11), 470–481.

Cato, C., Olson, D. K., & Studer, M. (1989). Incidence, prevalence, and variables associated with low back pain in staff nurses. *AAOHN Journal, 37*(8), 21–27.

Collins, J. W., Wolf, L., Bell, J., Evanoff, B. (2004). An evaluation of a "best practices" musculoskeletal injury prevention program in nursing homes. *Injury Prevention, 10*, 206–211.

Committee of the Connecticut Training-School for Nurses (1906). *A hand-book of nursing, revised edition: For hospital and general use.* Philadelphia: J.B. Lippincott Company.

Cust, G., Pearson, J., & Mair, A. (1972). The prevalence of low back pain in nurses. *International Nursing Review, 19*(2), 169–179.

Dehlin, O., & Lindberg, B. (1976). Back symptoms in nursing aides in a geriatric hospital. *Scandinavian Journal of Rehabilitative Medicine, 8*, 47–53.

Dehlin, O., Berg, S., Anderson, G. B. J., & Grimby, G. (1981). Effect of physical training and ergonomic counseling on the psychological perception of work and on the subjective assessment of low-back insufficiency. *Scandinavian Journal of Rehabilitative Medicine, 13*, 1–9.

Fash, B. (1946). *Body mechanics in nursing arts.* New York: McGraw-Hill Book Company, Inc.

Gagnon, M., Sicard, C., & Sirois, J. P. (1986). Evaluation of forces on the lumbosacral joint and assessment of work and energy transfers in nursing aides lifting patients. *Ergonomics, 29*(3), 407–421.

Garg, A. (1999). Long-term effectiveness of "zero-lift program" in seven nursing homes and one hospital. Contract No. U60/CCU512089-02. Accessed on October 25, 2004 at http://www.cdc.gov/nioshtic

Garg, A., & Owen, B. D. (1992). Reducing back stress to nursing personnel: an ergonomics intervention in a nursing home. *Ergonomics, 35*, 1353–1375.

Garg, A., Owen, B. D., & Carlson, B. (1992). An ergonomic evaluation of nursing assistants' job in a nursing home. *Ergonomics, 35*, 979–995.

Gill, H. Z. (1958). *Basic nursing* (4th ed.). New York: The Macmillan Company.

Goldman, R. H., Jarrard, M. R., Kim, R., Loomis, S., & Atkins, E. H. (2000). Prioritizing back injury risk in hospital employees: application and comparison of different injury rates. *Journal of Occupational and Environmental Medicine, 42*(6), 645–652.

Guo, H. R., Tanaka, S., Cameron, L. L., Seligman, P. J., Behrens, V. J., Ger, J., Wild, D. K., & Putz-Anderson, V. (1995). Back pain among workers in the United States: National estimates and workers at high risk. *American Journal of Industrial Medicine, 28*, 591–602.

Hampton, I. A. (1898). *Nursing: Its principles and practice.* Cleveland: J.B Savage.

Harber, P., Billet, E., Gutowski, M., SooHoo, K., Lew, M., & Roman, A. (1985). Occupational low-back pain in hospital nurses. *Journal of Occupational Medicine, 27*, 518–524.

Harber, P., Shimozake, S., Gargner, G., Billet, E., Vojtecky, M., & Kanim, L. (1987) Importance of non patient transfer activities in nursing-related back pain: II. Observational study and implications. *Journal of Occupational Medicine, 12*, 971–974.

Hawes, C. (1990). The Institute of Medicine study: Improving quality of care in nursing homes. In P. Katz, R. L. Kane, & M. Mezey (Eds.), *Advances in long-term care.* New York: Springer.

Health Resources and Services Administration, Bureau of Health Professions, National Center for Health Workforce Analysis (2002). *Projected supply, demand, and shortages of registered nurses: 2000–2020.* Retrieved May 20, 2004 from http://bhpr.hrsa.gov/healthworkforce/reports/rnproject/default.htm

Helminger, C. (1997). A growing physical workload threatens nurses' health. *American Journal of Nursing, 97,* 64–66.

Henderson, V. (1966). *The nature of nursing.* New York: Macmillan.

Institute of Medicine (1986). Improving the quality of care in nursing homes. Washington, D.C.: National Academy of Sciences Press.

Jensen, R. C. (1987). Disabling back injuries among nursing personnel: research needs and justification. *Research in Nursing and Health, 10*(1), 29–38.

Joel, L. A., & Kelly, L. Y. (2002). *The nursing experience: Trends, challenges, and transition.* New York: McGraw-Hill.

Klaber-Moffett, J. A., Hughes, G. I. & Griffiths, P. Z. (1993). A longitudinal study of low back pain in nurses. *International Journal of Nursing Studies, 30*(3), 197–212.

Klein, B., Jensen, R., & Sanderson, L. (1984). Assessment of worker's compensation claims for back strains/sprains. *Journal of Occupational Medicine, 26,* 443–448.

Lee, Y. H., & Chiou, W. K. (1994). Risk factors for low back pain, and patient handling capacity of nursing personnel. *Journal of Safety Research, 25*(3), 135–145.

Lipscomb, J. Trinkoff, A., Brady, B., & Geiger-Brown, J. (2004). Health care system changes and reported musculoskeletal disorders among registered nurses. *American Journal of Public Health, 94*(8), 1431–1435.

Lloyd, J. D. (2004). Biodynamics of back injury: Manual lifting and loads. In W. Charney, & A. Husdon (Eds.), *Back injury among healthcare workers: Causes, solutions, and impacts* (pp. 27–35). Boca Raton, FL: Lewis Publishers.

Marras, W. S., Davis, K. G., Kirking, B. C., & Bertsche, P. K. (1999). A comprehensive analysis of low-back disorder risk and spinal loading during the transferring and repositioning of patients using different techniques. *Ergonomics, 42,* 904–926.

Menzel, N. N. (1998). *Workers' comp from A to Z: A "how-to" book with forms.* Beverly Farms, MA: OEM Press.

Menzel, N. N. (2004). Back pain prevalence in nursing personnel. *AAOHN Journal, 52*(2), 54–65.

Menzel, N. N., Brooks, S. M., Bernard, T. E., & Nelson, A. (2004). The physical workload of nursing personnel: association with musculoskeletal discomfort. *International Journal of Nursing Studies, 41*(8), 859–867.

National Center for Health Statistics. *Health, United States, 2003.* Retrieved on May 20, 2004 from http://www.cdc.gov/nchs/data/hus/tables/2003/03hus090.pdf

National Council of State Boards of Nursing Examination Committee (2003). *National Council of State Boards of Nursing detailed test plan for the NCLEX-RN examination. Effective date April 2004.* Chicago: Author.

Needleman, J., Buerhaus, P., Mattke, S., Stewart, M., & Zelevinsky, K. (2002). Nurse-staffing levels and the quality of care in hospitals. *New England Journal of Medicine, 346,* 1715–1722.

Nelson, A., & Fragala, G. (2004). Equipment for safe patient handling and movement. In W. Charney, & A. Hudson (Eds.), *Back injury among health-*

care workers: Causes, solutions, and impacts (pp. 121–135). Boca Raton, FL: Lewis Publishers.

Nelson, A., Fragala, G., & Menzel, N. (2003a). Myths and facts about back injuries in nursing. *American Journal of Nursing, 103*(2), 32–40.

Nelson, A., Matz, M., Chen, F., Siddharthan, K., Lloyd, J., & Fragala, G. (2003b). Research report: A multifaceted ergonomics program to prevent injuries associated with patient handling tasks in the Veteran's Hospital Association.

Nurses have weak backs. (June 11, 1965). *Nursing Times,* 788–789.

Owen, B. D. (1987). The need for application of ergonomic principles in nursing. In S. S. Asfour (Ed.), Trends in ergonomics/human factors IV (pp. 831–838). North-Holland Elsevier Science Publishers, Amsterdam.

Owen, B. D. (1989). The magnitude of the low back problem in nursing. *Western Journal of Nursing, 11*(2), 234–242.

Owen, B. D., & Garg, A. (1991). Reducing risk for back pain in nursing personnel. *American Association of Occupational Health Nurses Journal, 39*(1), 24–33.

Personick, M. E. (1990, February). Nursing home aides experience increase in serious injuries. Bureau of Labor Statistics, *Monthly Labor Review.*

Pheasant, S., & Stubbs, D. (1992). Back pain in nurses: epidemiology and risk assessment. *Applied Ergonomics, 23*(4), 226–232.

Ronald, L. A., Yassi, A., Spiegel, J., Tate, R. B., Tait, D., & Mozel, M. R. (2002). Effectiveness of installing overhead ceiling lifts—reducing musculoskeletal injuries in an extended care hospital unit. *American Association of Occupational Health Nursing Journal, 50*(3), 120–127.

Sheldon, N. S., & Blodgett, J. B. (1946). Early rising in postoperative care. *American Journal of Nursing, 46*(6), 377–378.

Shogren, E., Calkins, A., & Wilburn, S. (1996). Restructuring may be hazardous to your health. *American Journal of Nursing, 96*(11), 64–66.

Smedley, J., Egger, P., Cooper, C., & Coggon, D. (1997). Prospective cohort study of predictors of incident low back pain in nurses. *British Medical Journal, 314* (7089), 1225–1228.

Snook, S. H., Campanelli, R. A., & Hart, J. W. (1978). A study of three preventive approaches to low back injury. *Journal of Occupational Medicine, 20,* 478–481.

Spiegel, J., Yassi, A., Ronald, L. A., Tate, R. B., Hacking, P., & Colby, T. (2002). Implementing a resident lifting system in an extended care hospital—demonstrating cost–benefit. *AAOHN Journal, 50*(3), 128–134.

Stubbs, D. A., Rivers, P., Hudson, M., & Worringham, C. (1981). Back pain research. *Nursing Times, 77,* 857–858.

Stubbs, D. A., Buckle, P. W., Hudson, M. P., Rivers, P. M., & Worringham, C. J. (1983). Back pain in the nursing profession: (1) epidemiology and pilot methodology. *Ergonomics, 26,* 755–766.

Svec, L. (1951, April). Oh, that aching back! *RN,* 30–32.

Tate, R. B., Yassi, A., Cooper, J. (1999). Predictors of time loss after back injury in nurses. *Spine, 24*(18), 1930–1935.

The nurse's load (editorial). (1965, August 28). *The Lancet,* ii, 422–423.

Tiesman, H., Nelson, A., Charney, W., Siddharthan, K., & Fragala, G. (2003). Effectiveness of a ceiling-mounted patient lift system in reducing occupational injuries in long-term care. *Journal of Healthcare Safety, 1*(1), 34–40.

Trinkoff, A. M., Lipscomb, J. A., Geiger-Brown, J., & Brady, B. (2002). Musculoskeletal problems of the neck, shoulder, and back and functional consequences in nurses. *American Journal of Industrial Medicine, 41*(3), 170–178.

Ulin, S. S., Chaffin, D. B., Patellow, C. L., Blitz, S. G., Emerick, C. A., Lundy, F., & Misher, L. (1997). A biomechanical analysis of methods used for transferring totally dependent residents. *SCI Nursing, 14*(1), 19–27.

US Department of Labor, Bureau of Labor Statistics (1994, June). *Worker safety problems spotlighted in health care industries. Summary 94–96.* Washington, DC: Author.

US Department of Labor, Bureau of Labor Statistics (2002). Standard occupational classification. Retrieved October 22, 2004, from http://www.bls.gov/soc

US Department of Labor, Bureau of Labor Statistics (2004). *Table 12. Number and median days of nonfatal occupational injuries and illnesses with days away from work involving musculoskeletal disorders by selected occupations, 2002.* Retrieved on June 2, 2004 from http://www.bls.gov/iif/oshwc/osh/case/ostb1267.pdf

Venning, P. J., Walter, S. D., Stitt, L. W. (1987). Personal and job-related factors as determinants of incidence of back injuries among nursing personnel. *Journal of Occupational Medicine, 29*(10), 820–825.

Videman, T., Nurminen, T., Tola, S., Kuorinka, I., Vanharanta, H., Troup, J. D. G. (1984). Low-back pain in nurses and some loading factors of work. *Spine, 9*(4), 400–404.

Waters, T., Putz-Anderson, V., Garg, A., & Fine, L. (1993). Revised NIOSH equation for the design and evaluation of manual lifting tasks. *Ergonomics, 36,* 749–776.

Winters, M. C. (1950). Nursing education: integration of body mechanics and posture in nursing. *American Journal of Nursing, 50*(11), 745–747.

Wood, D. J. (1986). Design and evaluation of a back injury prevention program within a geriatric hospital. *Spine, 12*(2), 77–82.

Wright, J. (1945). Protective body mechanics in convalescence. *American Journal of Nursing, 45*(9), 699–703.

Yassi, A., Khokhar, J., Tate, R., Cooper, J., Snow, C., & Vallentyne, S. (1995). The epidemiology of back injuries at a large Canadian tertiary care hospital: implications for prevention. *Occupational Medicine, 45*(4), 215–220.

Yassi, A., Cooper, J. E., Tate, R. B., Gerlach, S., Muir, M., Trottier, J., & Massey, K. (2001). A randomized controlled trial to prevent patient lift and transfer injuries of healthcare workers. *Spine, 26*(16), 1739–1746.

Zhuang, A., Stobbe, T. J., Hsiao, H., Collins, J. W., & Hobbs, G. R. (1999). Biomechanical evaluation of assistive devices for transferring residents. *Applied Ergonomics, 30,* 285–294.

CHAPTER TWO

Myths and Facts About Back Injuries in Nursing

Audrey L. Nelson, Guy Fragala, and Nancy N. Menzel

Hospitals and nursing homes have spent considerable time and effort attempting to prevent back injuries among nurses, with little improvement in the incidence or severity of musculoskeletal injuries. In 1989 there were 4.2 lost-workday injury and illness cases per 100 full-time workers in hospitals; in 2000 there were 4.1 per 100 (Bureau of Labor Statistics [BLS], n.d.). Healthcare institutions could undoubtedly use sound guidance in implementing more effective approaches to preventing injuries.

Manual lifting and other patient handling tasks are high-risk activities for both nurses and patients. The prevalence of work-related back injuries in nursing is among the highest of any profession internationally; annual prevalence rates of nursing-related back pain range from 35.9% in New Zealand (Coggan, Norton, Roberts, & Hope, 1994) to 47% in the United States (Trinkoff, Lipscomb, Geiger-Brown, & Brady, 2002) to 66.8% in the Netherlands (Knibbe & Friele, 1996). The 2000 incidence rate for back injuries involving days away from work was 181.6 per 10,000 full-time workers in nursing homes and 90.1 for hospitals, compared with incidence rates of 98.4 for truck drivers, 70 for

Reproduced with permission of the *American Journal of Nursing*, Vol. 103, No. 2, February 2003.

"The views expressed in this article are those of the authors and do not necessarily represent the view of the Department of Veterans Affairs. No claim made to U.S. government material. Contact Author: Audrey.Nelson@med.va.gov."

construction workers, 56.3 for miners, 47.1 for agricultural workers, and 43.2 for workers in manufacturing (BLS, n.d.). The rising rate of obesity also increases the risk of injury to nurses and other healthcare workers who handle patients. One of us (Menzel) studied patients in a Veterans Administration hospital and found that the weight of adult patients who required lifting ranged from 81 to 387 lbs. and averaged 169 lbs. The national nursing shortage intensified the need to protect nurses from injury. The time has come to abandon injury prevention strategies that have proved ineffective and to direct efforts to the following:

- Ergonomic assessment of patient care environments
- "Engineering controls" such as new ceiling-mounted mechanical lifting devices designed to reduce manual patient handling
- Standardized protocol for assessing the handling and moving of patients
- Algorithms for deciding about the number of personnel and type of equipment needed to handle and move patients safely
- A new education model that includes hospital-unit peer leaders who would ensure that workers use equipment competently and who could help change nursing practice

There are many misconceptions about how best to prevent musculoskeletal injuries when handling and moving patients. Countering the myths is the first step toward a solution.

MYTH

Education on Lifting Techniques and Training in Body Mechanics are Effective in Reducing Injuries

FACTS

Although it is widely accepted that classes in body mechanics and lifting techniques help to prevent job-related injuries, research in the past 35 years reveals that these efforts *by themselves* have consistently failed to reduce job-related injuries in healthcare as well as in other occupations (Brown, 1972; Buckle, 1987; Daltroy et al., 1997; Daws, 1981; Dehlin, Hedenrud, & Horal, 1976; Harber et al., 1994; Hayne, 1984; Lagerstrom & Hagberg, 1997; Owen & Garg, 1991; Snook, Campanelli & Hart, 1978; Stubbs, Buckle, Hudson, Rivers, & Worringham, 1983a; Stubbs, Buckle, Hudson, & Rivers, 1983b; Venning, 1988).

Education and training alone are not effective for several reasons. While nurses have been taught "proper" body mechanics for years, only recently have they begun to question whether the existing research on body mechanics can be safely applied to nursing. Early studies focused on men, and nursing still consists primarily of women. Research on lifting techniques should consider the effects of physical differences among nurses, for example the differences of upper-body strength in men and women.

People in early studies of body mechanics were asked to lift a box with handles—a task significantly easier than lifting a patient, whose mass is asymmetric, bulky, and cannot be held close to the body. Furthermore, patients can be combative, experience muscle spasms, or suddenly lose their balance; and a patient's ability to assist varies over the course of a day, making the same task different each time. The environment adds to the complexity; access to patients can be difficult because of bedside clutter or confinements of space, as in a bathroom, forcing nurses into awkward positions when assisting patients. Further research is needed into the effects of the nurse's sex and physique, the patient's weight, and the healthcare setting before the science of body mechanics can be fully applied to nursing practice.

To date, training in lifting techniques has been of limited value in healthcare settings. Because of differences among nurses, physical therapists, and exercise physiologists, experts do not always agree on the best ways for nurses to lift or assist dependent patients (Owen, 1985). Proponents of various lifting techniques have often failed to consider the following issues:

While biomechanical loading (forces applied to the body when performing a task) associated with lifting primarily involves the lower back, other body parts—particularly the knees and the shoulders—are quite vulnerable and may be injured as a result of the repeated lifting of heavy loads (Gagnon, Chehade, Kemp, & Lortie, 1987).

Balance often is not considered when nurses are taught to lift loads from below flexed knees with the back straight.

Not all stressful patient handling tasks are lifts, but techniques have focused exclusively on this task (Owen & Garg, 1990). Investigations show that nurses spend 20%–30% of their time bent forward or with the trunk twisted during activities such as bathing, dressing, and undressing patients.

Training programs fail to consider that lifting, turning, and repositioning patients are frequently performed on a horizontal plane, such as a bed or stretcher, requiring the nurse to use the weaker muscles of the arms and shoulders as the primary lifting muscles, rather than the stronger muscles of the legs.

Even if experts agreed on the best lifting techniques, it is unlikely that a single approach would reduce injuries: teaching a proper manual lifting technique is an attempt to modify behavior, which can be difficult to achieve and maintain without long-term reinforcement.

Further, the quest for effective manual techniques may be of limited value because, according to recent biomechanical evaluations, forces exerted on the musculoskeletal system when nurses perform patient handling tasks are beyond reasonable limits and capabilities, regardless of the technique used to perform the task manuals (Nelson, Lloyd, Menzel, & Gross, 2003; Owen, Garg, & Jensen, 1992). We advocate using engineering solutions (such as patient lifts, friction-reducing devices, or transfer belts) to reduce the risk of injury.

MYTH

High-Risk Tasks in Nursing are Restricted to Lifting Patients

FACTS

As mentioned, lifting patients is not the only stressful task in nursing. Many tasks, such as feeding, bathing, or dressing a patient, may have to be performed while bent forward with the torso twisted. Also, high-risk tasks performed on a horizontal plane are common, including the lateral transfer of a patient from bed to stretcher or repositioning a patient in bed.

Owen and Garg (1990) identified 16 stressful patient handling tasks performed in nursing homes. The most stressful tasks, identified in rank order, include:

- Transferring a patient from toilet to chair
- Transferring a patient from chair to toilet
- Transferring a patient from chair to bed
- Transferring a patient from bed to chair
- Transferring a patient from bathtub to chair
- Transferring a patient from chair lift to chair
- Weighing a patient
- Lifting a patient in bed
- Repositioning a patient from side to side in bed
- Repositioning a patient in a chair
- Changing an absorbent pad
- Making a bed with a patient in it

- Undressing a patient
- Tying supports
- Feeding a bedridden patient
- Making a bed without a patient in it

In an unpublished study, Nelson identified 10 stressful patient handing tasks in rehabilitation nursing, as follows (not in rank order):

- Bathing a patient in bed
- Making an occupied bed
- Dressing a patient in bed
- Transferring a patient from bed to Surgilift (Sunrise Medical, Longmont, Colorado)
- Transferring a patient from bed to stretcher
- Transferring a patient from bed to wheelchair
- Transferring a patient from bed to geri-chair
- Pulling a patient up in a chair
- Pulling a patient up to the head of the bed
- Putting anti-embolism stockings on a patient

MYTH

Injuries to Nurses Can be Prevented by Careful Screening of Nurses Before Hiring

FACTS

Many studies have explored how nurses affect their own risk. The motivation for this research is that potential employees might be screened or assigned to jobs according to their level of risk. Further, there is disagreement among researchers about which risk factors might be used to predict injuries. Factors to consider include level of fitness (Legg & Erg, 1987), obesity (Gold, 1994), genetics (Gold, 1994), height (Dehlin et al., 1976), muscular strength (Kilbom, 1988), age (Lavsky-Shulan et al, 1985), and stress (Hawkins, 1987). Restricting new hires to those without previous back injuries would make nursing recruitment almost impossible; nearly 87% of nurses report having had a back injury (Stubbs et al., 1983a,b; Fuortes, Shi, Zhang, Zwerling, & Schootman, 1994). In any case, such an approach may be discriminatory and illegal under the American with Disabilities Act.

Some behaviors and habits such as drug and alcohol consumption (Bigos et al, 1986; Manning, Libowitz, Goldberg, Rogers, & Newhouse, 1984) and cigarette smoking (Kelsey et al., 1984) might confound associations between occupation and a high risk of lower back pain. However, since many of these studies used correlational research designs (which do not examine causation), there is limited evidence about cause and effect between specific risk factors and musculoskeletal discomfort or injury.

MYTH

Back Belts are Effective in Reducing Risks to Caregivers

FACTS

Back belts have been used in many industries, including healthcare, to prevent musculoskeletal injuries, but there is no evidence that they are effective (Code of Federal Regulations (CFR), 2000).

Originally made of leather, back belts are now usually made of lightweight, breathable synthetic material and have at least one strap that tightens or loosens them. Supporters claim that such belts.

- Reduce internal forces on the spine when the back is forcefully exerted
- Increase intraabdominal pressure, which may counter the internal forces on the spine
- Stiffen the spine, which may decrease internal forces on the spine
- Restrict bending motions
- Remind the wearer to lift properly
- Reduce injuries in certain workplaces, such as those that require handling materials

According to a comprehensive study by the National Institute of Occupational Safety and Health (NIOSH), these claims remain unproved (NIOSH Back Belt Working Group, 1997). Lifting may produce a variety of forces within the body that contribute to loading (the pressure on the spine). The stresses created in the lower back when a person is handling materials manually are caused by the combination of the weight lifted and the method of handling the load—a combination that results in torque at various joints. The skeletal muscles are positioned to exert forces at these joints so that they counteract the torque. The excessive force generated by the lower back muscles is the primary source of compression forces on the lumbosacral discs. Because data indicate that the greatest problem is in the lower lumbar spine, many researchers consider stresses on the L5–S1 disk (lumbosacral joint) to be characteristic of the spinal stresses of lifting (NIOSH Back Belt Working Group, 1997).

Many of the studies NIOSH reviewed sought to examine the back belt's effect on loading, but none provided sufficient data to indicate that back belts significantly reduce loading during lifting. Some believe that the increased intraabdominal pressure thought to be provided by a back belt counterbalances loading forces on the spine, but this theory remains controversial. The studies on intraabdominal pressure that NIOSH reviewed were inconclusive, and its relationship to spinal compression is not well understood. Therefore, even if a back belt increased intraabdominal pressure, there is no evidence that it would reduce forces on the spine or decrease the risk of back injury.

Loading on the spine increases when a person bends farther forward. Some believe that if the back belt restricts the ability to bend, the risk of injury might be decreased. Although a back belt restricts range of motion during side-to-side bending and twisting, it does not have the same effect when a worker bends forward, as occurs when a nurse lifts a patient.

There is also no scientific evidence to support the claim that back belts remind workers to lift properly. But anecdotal case reports show a reduction in workplace injury when back belts have been used. Many companies that have instituted the use of belts have also installed new equipment and implemented programs in ergonomics, which may result in injury reduction. Based on available evidence, the back belts' capacity for reducing the occurrence of low back injuries remains unproved.

Some suggest that wearing a back belt may *increase* the potential for injury, because nurses may believe they can lift more while wearing a back belt. If they believe—erroneously—that they are protected, they may unwittingly increase their risk by trying to lift too much weight (NIOSH Back Belt Working Group, 1997).

MYTH

Various Lifting Devices are Equally Effective

FACTS

Use of some lifting devices can cause nearly as much stress to the musculoskeletal system as manual lifting does. Equipment should undergo ergonomic evaluation, and a proper device must be selected for the intended job. Whether nurses accept the equipment should also be determined. Numerous mechanical lifts, transfer devices, and lifting aids are available, and new products are always being developed. When considering mechanical lifts, there are two types: full-body sling lifts, which are normally used for a totally dependent patient; and stand-assist lifts, which are used for patients who have some weight-bearing capacity.

Full-body sling lifts may be mounted on a portable base or an overhead ceiling tracks. Both types have advantages. Portable-base units offer flexibility and can be moved from room to room as needed. Ceiling-mounted lifts are less convenient, but they do have one major advantage: nurses do not have to go looking for them when they are needed. Stand-assist lifts have simpler sling devices that take less time to put on, but their application is limited to patients with weight-bearing capacity, who can follow directions, and who are cooperative.

Methods of transfer other than sling lifts might be considered for totally dependent patients. A bed-to-chair transfer might be accomplished by using a chair that can bend back into a stretcher configuration, making this transfer more easily accomplished (Williamson et al., 1988). The transfer process can be further facilitated with a lateral-assist device, which can be powered electrically to pull the patient from the bed to the stretcher surface, or the device can be manual, such as a friction-reducing device with handles.

Vendors are eager to show their products, and demonstrations can easily be scheduled to properly evaluate equipment. Institutions should let nurses try these lift-assist devices so that they can determine which would be the most effective.

MYTH

Use of Mechanical Lifts Eliminates the Risks Involved in Manual Lifting

FACTS

Mechanical lifts can minimize the risk of injury but may not eliminate it. As previously discussed, there are high-risk tasks other than lifting, such as repositioning a patient, and often when using lifting equipment the patient must be lifted manually first so that the sling can be inserted. Also human effort is needed to move, guide, steady, and position the patient during the movement or transfer process.

Despite this, equipment that reduces the total burden of patient handling is highly beneficial since most injuries in nursing are due to cumulative trauma, that is, injuries occur slowly over time because of repeated musculoskeletal stress (Ronald et al., 2002). The key to reducing the risk of injury to nurses is to redesign high-risk lifting and handing tasks. A hierarchy of redesign strategies might be considered to accomplish this, as follows:

1. **Eliminate high-risk activities,** either by using equipment or delivering a service at the bedside instead of at a remote location. For example, beds that convert into chairs are available, thus eliminating the risks associated with manual bed-to-chair transfers. To eliminate the need to constantly reposition a patient in bed, a mattress that turns the patient from side to side can be used.
2. **Redesign high-risk tasks** to reduce some degree of risk. For example, use a mechanical lifting device to transfer a patient from bed to chair, minimizing the risk associated with manual lifting. While mechanical lifting devices may not eliminate the risk entirely, the cumulative reduction in effort may significantly reduce musculoskeletal discomfort and injuries.
3. **Choose alternative devices** to reduce the magnitude of risk. For example, if a mechanical lift to transfer a patient from bed to chair is not appropriate, a gait belt can be fastened around the patient's waist. (The belt can be secured by Velcro fasteners, and handles can be placed in a variety of configurations so that the caregiver can have better access to and control of a patient). Another option is a sling board that can bridge the bed and the chair so that the patient can slide in a seated position rather than being lifted.

MYTH

Mechanical Lifts are Not Affordable

FACTS

The costs of proper equipment are far lower than those associated with nurses' work-related injuries (Spiegel et al., 2002). In nine case studies that evaluated the use of lifting equipment in healthcare facilities, the incidence of injuries was reduced by 60%–95%, workers' compensation costs deceased by 95%, insurance premiums dropped by as much as 50%, medical and indemnity costs decreased by 92%, lost workdays (absence related to reported injury) decreased by as much as 100%, and absenteeism (absence related to unreported injury) was reduced by 98% (Fragala, 1993). As these studies show, lifting devices benefit the facility and nursing staff and also improve the quality of care given.

MYTH

If You Buy Lifting Equipment Staff Will Use It

FACTS

Administrators who purchase equipment are often frustrated when staff members do not use it and it ends up stored in a back room. Staff members have many reasons for not using equipment, including lack of time and availability, difficulty of use, space constraints, and patient preferences.

There are several ways to purchase costly equipment most efficiently. By including nursing staff in the selection process (Nelson, 2001), perhaps through an equipment fair or small clinical trial, facilities may improve staff acceptance.

Another common mistake is to purchase manually operated equipment rather than the slightly more expensive powered versions. According to our unpublished research with colleagues at the James A. Haley Veteran's Administration Hospital in Tampa, Florida, when deciding whether to use a lifting device, nurses compare the effort necessary to manually lift a patient with the extra time required to find and use lifting equipment. Minimizing obstacles can help increase the number of caregivers who use the equipment.

According to our research, other common mistakes include purchasing devices in insufficient quantities, putting the lifts in inconvenient locations, or inadequately maintaining equipment. When purchasing equipment, consider the ways in which nurses organize their assignments. Patient lifting is not evenly distributed throughout the day. Often, there are peak periods in which staff must compete for lifting devices, and few facilities have adequate and conveniently located storage space. It is critical to develop a successful plan for placing and maintaining equipment, including motor and frame upkeep, cleaning, laundering of slings, and sling and battery replacement.

MYTH

If You Simply Write a No-Lift Policy, Nurses Will Stop Lifting

FACTS

A few US hospitals have tried to institute a no-lift policy based on a successful policy in the United Kingdom. There, lifting devices have been provided by the National Health Service since 1983, and nurses are prohibited from lifting patient in routine situations, which significantly decreases the number of job-related injuries. The policy states that hazardous manual-handling tasks are to be avoided wherever possible; when unavoidable, they must be identified in advance and staff members must take action to remove or reduce the risk of injury. The policy further requires that facilities provide lifting equipment to nursing staff and other caregivers. Before any moving or handling procedure can be performed, the nurse should conduct a full risk assessment, completing the appropriate documentation (Manual Handling Operations Regulations, 1992).

Although administrators are often enamored of the idea, most attempts to implement no-lift policies in US hospitals have failed because they overlook technologic components. Infrastructure, including an adequate number of lifting devices, must first be in place in order to implement a successful no-lift policy, which must be focused on creating a safe workplace for caregivers, rather than on instituting punitive responses to mistakes (Plog & Quinlan, 2002).

EMERGING STRATEGIES

Several emerging technologies and strategies can improve nursing safety for both patients and nurses, based on engineering and administrative controls (Plog & Quinlan, 2002).

Engineering controls focus on bringing the activity to the patient rather than the reverse and substituting a lower risk task (such as a lateral transfer) for a higher risk once (such as a transfer from bed to chair) through the use of newer equipment.

Administrative controls focus on how nursing practice is performed, as well as how nurses are trained. While education in body mechanics and training in lifting techniques have been largely ineffective, a new educational model that takes advantage of peer leaders shows promise.

The Veterans Health Administration calls these peer leaders "back injury resource nurses" or BIRNs. An ongoing NIOSH study in a private healthcare facility refers to such peer leaders as "Ergo Rangers." These programs use a "train-the-trainer" approach to build a cadre of leaders who change nursing practice by teaching co-workers how to use equipment, advocating the use of assessment protocols and algorithms, reinforcing the use of practices such as adjusting bed height to a level that is comfortable for the nurse, and conducting ergonomic assessments of care environments (see the website of the Patient Safety Center of Inquiry at http://www.patientsafetycenter.com). Nelson and colleagues have developed patient assessment criteria and algorithms for safe patient handling and movement.

REFERENCES

Bigos, S., Spengler, D., Martin, N., Zeh, J., Fisher, L., Nachemson, A., & Wang, M. H. (1986). Back injuries in industry: a retrospective study. II. Injury factors. *Spine, 11*(3), 246–251.

Brown, J. (1972). *Manual lifting and related fields: An annotated bibliography.* Ottawa: Labor Safety Council of Ontario.

Buckle, P. (1987). Epidemiological aspects of back pain within the nursing profession. *International Journal of Nursing Studies, 24*(4), 319–324.

Bureau of Labor Statistics (BLS) (2002). *Occupational industries and illnesses: Industry data.* Retrieved May 2, 2005, from http://www.bls.gov/data/archived.htm

Code of Federal Regulations (2000). *Title 29, Part 1910.* Washington, DC: Government Printing Office.

Coggan, C., Norton, R., Roberts, I., & Hope, V. (1994). Prevalence of back pain among nurses. *New Zealand Medical Journal, 107*(983), 306–308.

Daltroy, L. H., Iversen, M. D., Larson, M. G., Lew, R., Wright, E., Ryan, J., Zwerling, C., Fossel, A. H., & Liang, M. H. (1997). A controlled trial of an educational program to prevent low back injuries. *The New England Journal of Medicine, 337*(5), 322–328.

Daws, J. (1981). Lifting and moving patients. 3. A revision training programme. *Nursing Times, 77*(48), 2067–2069.

Dehlin, O., Hedenrud, B., & Horal, J. (1976). Back symptoms in nursing aides in a geriatric hospital. An interview study with special reference to the incidence of low-back symptoms. *Scandinavian Journal of Rehabilitation Medicine, 8*(2), 47–53.

Fragala, G. (1993). Injuries cut with lift use in ergonomics demonstration project. *Provider 19*(10), *October,* 39–40.

Fuortes, L. J., Shi, Y., Zhang, M., Zwerling, C., & Schootman, M. (1994). Epidemiology of back injury in university hospital nurses from review of workers compensation records and a case-control survey. *Journal of Occupational Medicine, 36*(9), 1022–1026.

Gagnon, M., Chehade, A., Kemp, F., & Lortie, M. (1987). Lumbo-sacral loads and selected muscle activity while turning patients in bed. *Ergonomics, 30*(7), 1013–1032.

Gold, M. (1994). The ergonomic workplace: charting a course for long-term care. *Provider, 20*(2), 20–23, 26.

Harber, P., Pena, L., Hsu, P., Billet, E., Greer, D., & Kim, K. (1994). Personal history, training, and worksite as predictors of back pain of nurses. *American Journal of Industrial Medicine, 25*(4), 519–526.

Hawkins, L. (1987). An ergonomic approach to stress. *International Journal of Nursing Studies, 24*(4), 307–318.

Hayne, C. (1984). Ergonomics and back pain. *Physiotherapy, 70*(1), 9–13.

Kelsey, J. L., Githens, P. B., White, A. A. III, Holford, T. R., Walter, S. D., O'Connor, T., Ostfeld, A. M., Weil, U., Southwick, W. O., & Calogero, J. A. (1984). An epidemiologic study of lifting and twisting on the job and risk for acute prolapsed lumbar intervertebral disc. *Journal of Orthopaedic Research, 2*(1), 61–66.

Kilbom, A. (1988). Isometric strength and occupational muscle disorders. *European Journal of Applied Physiology and Occupational Physiology, 57*(3), 322–326.

Knibbe, J. J., & Friele, R. D. (1996). Prevalence of back pain and characteristics of the physical workload of community nurses. *Ergonomics, 39*(2), 186–198.

Lagerstrom, M., & Hagberg, M. (1997). Evaluation of a 3-year education and training program for nursing personnel at a Swedish hospital. *AAOHN Journal, 45*(2), 83–92.

Lavsky-Shulan, M., Wallace, R. B., Kohout, F. J., Lemke, J. H., Morris, M. C., & Smith, I. M. (1985). Prevalence and functional correlates of low back pain in the elderly: the Iowa 65+ Rural Health Study. *Journal of the American Geriatrics Society, 33*(1), 23–28.

Legg, S., & Erg, S. (1987). Physiological ergonomics in nursing. *International Journal of Nursing Studies, 24*(4), 299–305.

Manning, W. G., Leibowitz, A., Goldberg, G. A., Rogers, W. H., & Newhouse, J. P. (1984). A controlled trial of the effect of a prepaid group practice on use of services. *New England Journal of Medicine, 310*(23), 1505–1510.

Manual Handling Operations Regulations (1992). SI 1992/2793.

Nelson, A. L. (Ed.). (2001). *Patient care ergonomics resource guide: Safe patient handling and movement.* Retrieved May 3, 2005, from http://www.patientsafetycenter.com/Safe%20Pt%20Handling%20Div.htm

Nelson, A. L., Lloyd, J., Menzel, N., & Gross, C. (2003). Preventing nursing back injuries: redesigning patient handling tasks. *AAOHN Journal, 51*(3), 126–134.

NIOSH Back Belt Working Group (1997). *Workplace use of back belts: Review and recommendations.* Rockville, MD: National Institute for Occupational Safety and Health.

Owen, B. D. (1985). The lifting process and back injury in hospital nursing personnel. *Western Journal of Nursing Research, 7*(4), 445–459.

Owen, B., & Garg, A. (1990). Assistive devices for use with patient handling tasks. In B. Das (Ed.), *Advances in industrial ergonomics and safety.* Philadelphia, PA: Taylor & Frances.

Owen, B., & Garg, A. (1991). Reducing risk for back pain in nursing personnel. *AAOHN Journal, 39*(1), 24–33.

Owen, B., Garg, A., & Jensen, R. C. (1992). Four methods for identification of most back-stressing tasks performed by nursing assistants in nursing homes. *International Journal of Industrial Ergonomics, 9,* 213–220.

Plog, B., & Quinlan, P. J. (Eds.). (2002). *Fundamentals of industrial hygiene* (5th ed.). Itasca, IL: National Safety Council.

Ronald, L. A., Yassi, A., Spiegel, J., Tate, R. B., Tait, D., & Mozel, M. R. (2002). Effectiveness of installing overhead ceiling lifts. *AAOHN Journal, 50*(3), 120–126.

Spiegel, J., Tassi, A., Ronald, L. A., Tate, R. B., Hacking, P., & Colby, T. (2002). Implementing a resident lifting system in an extended care hospital. *AAOHN Journal, 50*(3), 128–134.

Snook, S., Campanelli, R., & Hart, J. (1978). A study of three preventative approaches to low back injury. *Journal of Occupational Medicine, 20*(7), 478–481.

Stubbs, D. A., Buckle, P., Hudson, M. P., Rivers, P. M., & Worringham, C. J. (1983a). Back pain in the nursing profession. I. Epidemiology and pilot methodology. *Ergonomics, 26*(8), 755–765.

Stubbs, D. A., Buckle, P., Hudson, M. P., & Rivers, P. M. (1983b). Back pain in the nursing profession. II. The effectiveness of training. *Ergonomics, 26*(8), 767–779.

Trinkoff, A. M., Lipscomb, J. A., Geiger-Brown, J., & Brady, B. (2002). Musculoskeletal problems of the neck, shoulder, and back and functional consequences in nurses. *American Journal of Industrial Medicine, 41*(3), 170–178.

Venning, P. (1988). Back injury prevention among nursing personnel. *AAOHN Journal, 36*(8), 327–333.

Williamson, K., Turner, J., Brown, K., Newman, K., Sirles, A., & Selleck, C. (1988). Occupational health hazards for nurses, part 2. *Image—The Journal of Nursing Scholarship, 20*(3), 162–168.

CHAPTER THREE

Consequences of Unsafe Patient Handling Practices

Audrey L. Nelson

Despite the convincing argument in Chapter 1 that patient handling tasks are high-risk tasks frequently resulting in injuries to the patient and the caregiver, many patient care providers, managers, and administrators fail to appreciate the danger and are slow to implement evidence-based interventions to promote safe patient handling and movement. Others espouse support for safer work environments, but subtly undermine safety initiatives through an organizational culture that emphasizes productivity goals over those of safety. Injuries are likely to occur in these environments where there are constant tradeoffs between speed versus accuracy, or safety versus production (Moray, 1994). As an example, workload pressures force nursing staff to cut corners (e.g., manually lift a patient rather than search for a lifting device) in order to get assignments completed in a timely fashion. The purpose of this chapter is to describe the far-reaching consequences of unsafe patient handling practices for the injured nurse, the patient, and the organization.

"The views expressed in this article are those of the author and do not necessarily represent the view of the Department of Veterans Affairs. No claim made to U.S. government material. Contact Author: Audrey.Nelson@med.va.gov."

CONSEQUENCES FOR THE INJURED NURSE

The person most likely to suffer the consequences of unsafe patient handling practices is the direct care provider. These unintended consequences go beyond the significant numbers and severity of injuries, and include (1) guilt and blame for the injury, (2) chronic pain and a fear of reinjury or permanent disability, (3) deleterious impact on quality of life, and (4) unwanted career changes. Each will be briefly described.

Guilt and Blame for the Injury

The injured nurse faces guilt and may blame him/herself or find others blaming him/her for the injury. There is a fundamental need to assign blame when an injury occurs, based on (a) "fundamental attribution error," a tendency to identify weaknesses of the person who was injured as a way to rationalize why the injury occurred; (b) "illusion of free will," where we believe people are in control of their actions, despite hazards that are evident in the workplace; and (c) "similarity bias," which convinces us that there is more order in the world than actually exists, rationalizing why this would not happen to us (Reason, 1994).

When an injury occurs, the nurse may blame him/herself for transitory mental states associated with errors, such as momentary inattention, distraction, or preoccupation, despite the fact that these are the last and least manageable links in the error chain because they are unintended and largely unpredictable (Reason, 1994).

Other nursing staff on a unit may harbor resentment when an injured caregiver reports an injury. While on the surface this appears to be cruel and unfeeling, often this resentment may emerge from a sense of self-preservation, since patient handling injuries are most often cumulative in nature, the injured caregiver often performs for days or weeks with increasing severity and duration of musculoskeletal discomfort. This discomfort is likely due to heavy patient care demands which also affect the other caregivers on the unit, who also have musculoskeletal discomfort of increasing severity and duration. Often injured workers are not replaced, which means the remaining staff share the injured worker's workload, increasing their own exposure to risk.

Chronic Pain and a Fear of Reinjury or Permanent Disability

Most care providers suffer from significant musculoskeletal discomfort that can last days or weeks at a time. Frequently, this discomfort goes unreported until it interferes with the performance of job tasks. Even when the injured worker is treated and takes time off to heal, he/she may face chronic pain and discomfort at the end of each shift. The injured care provider may also fear he/she will be reinjured once back to duty. Chronic musculoskeletal discomfort and a fear of reinjury (Dillman, 1994) may lead to tentativeness in the way patient handling tasks are performed or avoidance of many high-risk tasks to prevent permanent disability.

Deleterious Impact on Quality of Life

Injured nurses have impaired quality of life associated with chronic pain or functional impairments. Many find that their work-related musculo-skeletal discomfort interferes with their leisure time activities.

Unwanted Career Changes

Injured caregivers may also worry that the injury could negatively affect their career. For example, a serious injury could result in the need to transfer to another nursing position where patient handling demands are less, or may necessitate an unwanted career change away from patient care altogether, either temporarily or permanently. This may also lead to concern about how their injury could affect career prospects in the future (Wicker, 2000).

CONSEQUENCES FOR THE PATIENT

There are significant clinical consequences of unsafe patient handling as well, including the impact on (1) quality of care and (2) patient comfort and safety (Wicker, 2000). Each will be briefly described.

Quality of Care

In many cases injured nurses are not replaced when they are away from work or on restricted duty, creating staff shortages, which detract from patient care quality. Further, nurses with significant musculoskeletal pain or those on modified duty may not be physically able to get patients out of bed as frequently or perform other physically demanding tasks, essentially decreasing patient services by default. One of the most physically demanding task is a patient transfer out of bed. There is a long list of patient adverse events associated with prolonged bed rest, including toileting problems/incontinence, pressure ulcers, falls, contractures, deep vein thrombosis, acute confusional states, decline in functional status, and pneumonia.

Patient Comfort and Safety

When an injured nurse attempts to perform patient handling tasks with limited strength or musculoskeletal pain, the results can include resident discomfort (US Department of Labor, 2002) or adverse events associated with dropping patients, dragging patients across surfaces, or frightening patients with jerky movements during transfer tasks. Patients can respond to these practices with fear, and may suffer pain, damage to shoulder, hip fractures, bruises, increased dependency, skin tears, pressure area damage, or loss of dignity during lifting procedure. (Tuohy-Main, 1997).

CONSEQUENCES FOR THE ORGANIZATION

There are significant organizational level consequences of unsafe patient handling as well, including the impact on (1) productivity, (2) recruitment and retention of caregivers, and (3) costs. Each will be briefly described.

Productivity

Work-related musculoskeletal injuries in nursing have serious consequences to the organization. A loss of productivity results from absenteeism (US Department of Labor, 2002), lost or modified workdays (Dillman, 1993), and the difficulties imposed with scheduling and coverage on affected nursing units. The cumulative effect of nursing injuries can lead to staff shortages (Dillman, 1993) and permanent loss of experienced nursing staff to disability or decision to leave the job (Corlett, Lloyd, Tarling, Troup, & Wright, 1993).

Recruitment and Retention of Nurses

Recruitment and retention of nurses is a serious problem, exacerbated by nurses with job-related injuries. In one survey of injured nurses, 12% of respondents indicated they were considering making an employment transfer and another 12% said they were thinking of leaving the nursing profession due to back pain (Owen, 1989). A study in England found that 12% of nurses who intended to leave nursing permanently cited back pain as a main or contributing factor (Stubbs, 1986). A third study in 1992 queried 99,955 RNs who left the profession; 18.3% said it was because of concern for safety in the healthcare environment (Moses, 1992).

Organizational Costs

Another organizational concern is the significant costs associated with injuries to care providers (Dillman, 1993; US Department of Labor, 2002). In addition to the direct costs of medical treatment and compensation, the organization faces hidden factors that inflate the average claim loss by a factor of five, including temporary hires for replacement personnel, overtime to absorb the duties of injured worker, legal fees; time loss costs for claim processing, witnesses; decreased output following traumatic event; training temporary and/or replacement personnel (Charney, Zimmerman, & Walara, 1991; US Department of Labor, 2002). Organizations may be concerned about the risk of liability (Corlett et al., 1993; Wicker, 2000) as well as regulatory deficiencies associated with hazardous work environments. Lastly, the organization can face the effects of diminished staff morale and job satisfaction (US Department of Labor, 2002), exacerbating the serious problems associated with recruitment and retention of nurses.

Given the high incidence and prevalence of work-related musculoskeletal injuries associated with caregiving, it is not surprising that their associated costs are also significant. In 1990, the estimated cost of back pain ranged from $50 to $100 billion annually in the United States (Frymoyer & Cats-Baril, 1991). Employee turnover, reduced production, and medical cost reimbursement are estimated at an additional $30 billion annually. Back pain is second to only the common cold as the most frequent cause for sick leave (Klein, Jensen, & Sanderson, 1984; US Department of Labor, 1992) and is the most common reason for filing of workers' compensation claims.

SUMMARY

The goal of healthcare is to continually reduce the burden of illness, injury, and disability, and to improve the health and functioning of the patients who seek medical advice (Institute of Medicine, 2001). Unsafe working environments jeopardize this goal, through unintended adverse consequences for the patient, care provider, and the organization. Unsafe patient handling can actually potentiate patient illness or injury, impede patient functional status, interfere with patient healing, and compromise patient safety. They can also result in deleterious effects on the caregiver, potentially jeopardizing his/her nursing career. The organization suffers significant financial loss in both production costs and workers' compensation costs, and may find barriers imposed for recruiting and retaining a competent nursing staff.

REFERENCES

Charney, W., Zimmerman, K., & Walara, E. (1991). The lifting team: a design method to reduce lost time back injury in nursing. *AAOHN Journal, 39*(5), 231–234.

Corlett, E. N., Lloyd, P. V., Tarling, C., Troup, J. D. G., & Wright, B. (1993). *The guide to handling patients* (3rd ed.). London: National Back Pain Association and the Royal College of Nursing.

Dillman, S. (1994). An ergonomic approach to the prevention of back injuries in the healthcare industry. 1993 AHEHP Conference, Presentation by Guy Fragala. *Journal of Hospital Occupational Health, 13*(3), 13–15.

Frymoyer, J. W., & Cats-Baril, W. L. (1991). An overview of the incidences and costs of low back pain. *Orthopaedic Physical Therapy Clinics of North America, 22*(2), 263–271.

Institute of Medicine (2001). *Crossing the quality chasm* (p. 6). Washington, DC: National Academy Press.

Klein, B. P., Jensen, R. C., & Sanderson, L. M. (1984). Assessment of workers' compensation claims for back strains/sprains. *Journal of Occupational Medicine, 26*(6), 443–448.

Moray, N. (1994). Error reduction as a systems problem. In M. S. Bogner (Ed.), *Human error in medicine* (pp. 67–91). Hillsdale, NJ: Lawrence Erlbaum Associates.

Moses, E. B. (Ed.). (1992). *The registered nurse population: Findings from the national sample survey of registered nurses* (p. 65). Washington, DC: US Department of Human Services, US Public Health Service, Division of Nursing #5.

Owen, B. D. (1989). The magnitude of low-back problems in nursing. *Western Journal of Nursing Research, 11*(2), 234–242.

Reason, J. T. (1994). Forward. In M. S. Bogner (Ed.), *Human error in medicine.* Hillsdale, NJ: Lawrence Erlbaum Associates.

Stubbs, D. (1986). Backing out: nurse wastage associated with back pain. *International Journal of Nursing Studies, 23*(4), 325–336.

Tuohy-Main, K. (1997). Why manual handling should be eliminated for resident and career safety. *Geriatrician, 15*, 10–14.

US Department of Labor, Occupational Safety and Health Administration (2002). Ergonomics Guidelines for Nursing Homes. Retrieved April 18, 2005, from http://www.osha.gov/ergonomics/guidelines/nursinghome/final_nh_guidelines.html

Wicker, P. (2000). Manual handling in the perioperative environment. *British Journal of Perioperative Nursing, 10*(5), 255–259.

Variations in High-Risk Patient Handling Tasks by Practice Setting

Audrey L. Nelson

While physical environment, work practices, and safety culture influence which ergonomic interventions to implement, key to understanding the inherent risks associated with each clinical setting is the number, type, and frequency of each high-risk task performed. The purpose of this chapter is to characterize high-risk tasks across clinical settings, as a precursor to designing appropriate ergonomic solutions.

DEFINITION OF HIGH-RISK PATIENT HANDLING TASKS

High-risk patient handling tasks are defined as duties that impose significant biomechanical and postural stressors on the care provider (Nelson, Lloyd, Menzel, & Gross, 2003). Several contributing factors influence

"The views expressed in this article are those of the authors and do not necessarily represent the view of the Department of Veterans Affairs. No claim made to U.S. government material. Contact Author: Audrey.Nelson@med.va.gov."

the level of risk, including the patient's weight, transfer distance, confined workspace and aspects of the physical environment, unpredictable patient behavior, availability of technological solutions, and awkward positions such as stooping, bending, and reaching. The frequency and duration of these tasks also influence the threat to caregiver safety. For example, it is wise to focus on high-risk tasks that are performed frequently rather than to design a solution for a high-risk task performed less than once per week. Further, more efforts need to be made for re-designing high-risk tasks of long duration, as these are likely to be more strenuous and risky for the caregivers. Examples of tasks of long duration include feeding a confused bedridden patient or providing a bed bath to a patient.

Few would argue that one of the highest risk tasks associated with patient handling is a manual patient transfer. Patient transfers can start with the patient in a sitting position (vertical transfer) or when the patient is supine (lateral transfer) (Nelson & Fragala, 2004). However, not all high-risk tasks involve patient transfers. Other high-risk patient handling tasks include repositioning a patient in bed, repositioning a patient in a chair, and transporting a patient in a bed or stretcher. Further, risk for injury extends beyond tasks that involve patient movement. Patient handling tasks can be designated as high risk if they are performed in a forwardly bent position with the torso twisted, such as feeding, bathing, or dressing a patient.

It is the combination of frequency and duration of these high-risk tasks that predispose a caregiver to musculoskeletal injuries, and make some clinical practice settings more dangerous than others (Nelson et al., 2004).

High-risk tasks push the limits of human capabilities, contributing to either acute or cumulative trauma. The following characteristics have been defined for high-risk tasks:

- Heavy loads
- Sustained awkward positions
- Bending and twisting
- Reaching
- Fatigue or stress
- Force
- Standing for long periods of time

Hignett et al. (2003) summarized available evidence published before 2003 to create an evidence base for high-risk tasks. They found that there was a moderate level of evidence to support three patient handling tasks as high risk:

1. Hazardous tasks involve moving patients in bed, bed–chair transfers, toileting, bathing, and lifting from the floor (Bell, Dalgity, Fennell, & Aitken, 1979; Garg, Owen, & Carlson, 1992; Hui, Ng, Yeung, & Hui-Chan, 2001; Owen 1987; Owen, Garg, & Jensen, 1992; Schibye & Skotte, 2000; Smedley, Egger, Cooper, & Coggon, 1995).
2. Ambulance work can result in harmful postures, with the highest risks involving the transportation of patients on equipment (Doormaal, Driessen, Landeweerd, & Drost, 1995; Furber, Moore, Williamson, & Barry, 1997; Massad, Gambin, & Duval, 2000).
3. A high-risk task for home care nursing is providing care in non-adjustable beds (Ballard, 1994; Knibbe & Friele, 1996; Skarplik, 1988).

DEFINING PRACTICE SETTINGS WHERE PATIENT HANDLING TASKS ARE PERFORMED

Patient handling tasks are performed across in a variety of settings, including inpatient, outpatient, and community-based settings. These tasks are performed across the care continuum, including acute care, specialty care, long-term care, and home care. Caregivers provide services across the age continuum, including pediatric, adult, and geriatric care. The types of patients in any given caseload also varies, and can be characterized by patient characteristics that affect patient handling and dependency levels, including functional impairments, cognition, and level of cooperation. Given the diversity in the settings and types of patients cared for, it is not surprising that the type, frequency, and duration of caregiving tasks vary widely. Units where there are a disproportionate number of physically dependent patients are likely to require larger number of high-risk patient handling tasks.

HIGH-RISK PATIENT HANDLING TASKS BY SETTING

Research related to segmenting specific high-risk task by practice setting is somewhat sparse. A better understanding of high-risk tasks by setting would promote the appropriate translation of evidence-based patient care ergonomic solutions. For the purpose of this chapter, evidence is available to identify high-risk tasks in the following settings:

1. Operating room
2. Medical/surgical

3. Psychiatry
4. Rehabilitation/spinal cord injury
5. Critical care units
6. Trauma/emergency
7. Long-term care
8. Home care

The evidence in each of these clinical settings will be briefly reviewed.

High-Risk Tasks in Operating Room (OR)

Owen in the United States (Owen, 2000) and Wicker in the United Kingdom (Wicker, 2000) identified high-risk tasks for OR nurses, including the following pre-, peri-, and post-operative tasks.

- Standing for long periods of time (Owen, 2000)
- Adopting unnatural positions in order to work effectively or leaning over the patient for protracted periods (Wicker, 2000)
- Lifting and holding patient's extremities (Owen, 2000) or prepping a limb (Wicker, 2000)
- Holding retractors for extended periods of time (Owen, 2000)
- Transferring patients on and off OR beds (Owen, 2000; Garb & Dockery, 1995)
- Reaching, lifting, and moving equipment (Owen, 2000; Garb & Dockery, 1995; Wicker, 2000)
- Repositioning patients in OR beds (Owen, 2000; Wicker, 2000)
- Slippery shoe covers and floors (Garb & Dockery, 1995)
- Tripping hazards (Garb & Dockery, 1995)

High-Risk Tasks in Medical/Surgical Units

While there were no specific studies that addressed high-risk tasks in medical/surgical units, the following tasks were generalized from "acute care:"

- Transfer from bed to chair
- Transfer from bed to stretcher
- Moving occupied bed or stretcher
- Making occupied bed
- Bathing a confused or totally dependent patient

- Lifting a patient up from the floor
- Weighing a patient
- Applying anti-embolism stockings
- Repositioning in bed
- Extensive dressing changes

High-Risk Tasks in Psychiatry Units

While there were no specific studies that addressed high-risk tasks in psychiatry units, the following tasks were identified. It is hypothesized that geriatric psychiatry units would have a higher concentration of high-risk tasks than other psychiatric units. Further research is needed in this area.

- Restraining a patient
- Escorting a confused or combative patient
- Toileting a confused or combative patient
- Dressing a confused or combative patient
- Picking a patient up from the floor
- Bathing/showering a confused or combative patient
- Bed-related care

High-Risk Tasks in Rehabilitation/Spinal Cord Injury Units

Nelson (1996) identified the following rehabilitation nursing tasks as high risk. It is the combination of a high number of physically dependent patients with a unit philosophy to get the patients dressed and out of bed on a daily basis that increases the risk to these caregivers.

- Transferring patient from toilet to chair
- Transferring patient from wheelchair to bed
- Repositioning a patient to the head of the bed, or side to side
- Repositioning a patient in a wheelchair
- Making an occupied bed
- Dressing/undressing a patient
- Feeding a bedridden patient
- Ambulating a patient at high risk for falls
- Showering a patient or providing a bed bath
- Applying anti-embolism stockings (TED hose)

High-Risk Tasks in Critical Care Units

Nelson (1996) conducted a pilot study to examine high-risk tasks in nine critical care units. Key tasks identified include:

- Transporting patients in bed or stretcher, frequently with heavy monitors and multiple lines (also known as "road trips")
- Lateral transfers (bed to stretcher)
- Lifting patient to the head of the bed
- Transferring patients on and off cardiac chairs
- Repositioning patient in bed from side to side
- Making an occupied bed
- Moving heavy equipment and accessing electrical outlets
- Providing patient handling tasks in crowded area, where multiple lines and monitoring equipment force caregivers into awkward positions
- Performing cardiopulmonary resuscitation or other procedures with the bed at a wrong height (many team members are present and it is impossible to have the bed at the right height for all the staff)
- Applying anti-embolism stockings

High-Risk Tasks in Trauma/Emergency

Little work has been done related to the high-risk tasks in trauma and emergency settings. A moderate level of evidence is available to support that ambulance work can result in harmful postures, with the highest risks involved in the transportation of patients on equipment (Doormaal et al., 1995; Furber et al., 1997; Massad et al., 2000). Patient transfers in and out of personal vehicles are also considered a high-risk task, particularly when the patient presents at the emergency room acutely ill. Unfortunately, this task has not been well studied.

High-Risk Tasks in Nursing Home or Long-Term Care Facilities

Owen and Garg (1990) identified 16 stressful patient handling tasks in nursing homes. Several other researchers have also examined risks in this setting (Garg et al., 1992; Hui et al., 2001; Nelson, 1998; Owen, 1987; Owen et al., 1992; Schibye & Skotte, 2000; Smedley et al., 1995). The most stressful tasks identified included:

- Transferring patient from toilet to chair
- Transferring patient from chair to toilet
- Transferring patient from chair to bed

- Transferring patient from bed to chair
- Transferring patient from bathtub to chair
- Transferring patient from chair lift to chair
- Weighing a patient
- Lifting a patient up in the bed
- Repositioning a patient in the bed side to side
- Repositioning a patient in a chair
- Changing an absorbent pad
- Making a bed with the patient in it
- Undressing a patient
- Tying supports
- Feeding a bedridden patient
- Making a bed while the patient is not in it

High-Risk Tasks in Home Care

A few researchers have explored high-risk tasks performed in home care (Ballard, 1994; Knibbe & Friele, 1996; Owen & Staehler, 2003; Skarplik, 1988). Home care offers unique challenges, since there is great variation and less than ideal working conditions.

- Providing patient care in a bed that is not height adjustable
- Providing care in a crowded area, forcing awkward positions
- Toileting and transfer tasks without proper lifting aids
- No assistance for tasks

STRATEGIES FOR ASSESSING HIGH-RISK TASKS

Through job observation, questionnaires to employees, or brainstorming sessions with patient handlers, individual sites should determine what are the high-risk activities within their workplace. Figure 4.1 is a tool that can be used by the nursing staff to identify and prioritize high-risk tasks. Keep in mind that there are variations likely to be of high-risk tasks by unit as well as by shift.

SUMMARY

Patient handling practices vary widely by clinical area. The first step in developing a patient care ergonomics program is to identify the unique high-risk tasks associated with practices on that specific work site. Once

Directions: Assign a rank (from 1 to 10) to the tasks you consider to be the highest risk tasks contributing to musculoskeletal injuries for persons providing direct patient care. A "1" should represent the highest risk, "2" for the second highest, etc. For each task, consider the frequency of the task (high, moderate, and low) and musculoskeletal stress (high, moderate, and low) of each task when assigning a rank. Delete tasks not typically performed on your unit. You can have each nursing staff member complete the form and summarize the data, or you can have staff work together by shift to develop the rank by consensus.

Frequency of task	Stress of task	Rank	Patient handling tasks
H, high; M, moderate; L, low	H, high; M, moderate; L, low	1, high risk; 10, low risk	
			Applying anti-embolism stockings
			Bathing patient in bed
			Bathing a patient in the tub
			Changing an absorbent pad
			Dressing/undressing a patient
			Feeding a bedridden patient
			Holding an arm or leg for extended periods (e.g., surgery or dressing changes)
			Holding retractors for extended periods of time
			Making an occupied bed
			Patient transfers in and out of personal vehicles
			Picking a patient up off the floor post-fall
			Providing care in non-height adjustable beds
			Repositioning a patient in a chair or wheelchair
			Repositioning a patient in the bed side to side
			Toileting a patient
			Transferring a patient from bed to stretcher
			Transferring a patient from bed to chair
			Transporting patient off unit
			Other task:
			Other task:
			Other task:

Adapted from Owen, B. D., & Garg, A. (1991). Reducing risk for back pain in nursing personnel. *AAOHN Journal, 39*(1), 24–33.

FIGURE 4.1 Tool for prioritizing high-risk patient handling tasks.

the high-risk tasks are identified, appropriate ergonomic solutions can be developed. Further research is needed related to (1) the most efficient and effective strategies to identify high-risk tasks related to patient care; (2) characterization of high-risk tasks by clinical setting, particularly in understudy areas such as trauma/emergency, medical/surgical, obstetrics, pediatrics, orthopedics, and bariatrics, as well as outpatient exam rooms, to name a few; and (3) linkage between specific high-risk tasks and ergonomic solutions.

REFERENCES

Ballard, J. (1994). District nurses—who's looking after them? *Occupational Health Review, Nov./Dec.,* 10–16.

Bell, F., Dalgity, M. E., Fennell, M. J., & Aitken, R. C. B. (1979). Hospital ward patient-lifting tasks. *Ergonomics, 22*(11), 1257–1273.

Doormaal, M., Driessen, A., Landeweerd, J., & Drost, M. R. (1995). Physical workload of ambulance assistants. *Ergonomics, 38*(2), 361–376.

Furber, S., Moore, H., Williamson, M., & Barry, J. (1997). Injuries to ambulance officers caused by patient handling tasks. *Journal of Occupational Health & Safety—Australia & New Zealand, 13*(3), 259–265.

Garb, J. R., & Dockery, C. A. (1995). Reducing employee back injuries in the perioperative setting. *AORN Journal, 61*(6), 1046–1052.

Garg, A., Owen, B., & Carlson, B. (1992). Ergonomic evaluation of nursing assistants' jobs in a nursing home. *Ergonomics, 35*(9), 979–995.

Hignett, S., Crumpton, E., Ruszala, S., Alexander, P., Fray, M., & Fletcher, B. (2003). *Evidence-based patient handling: Tasks, equipment and interventions.* New York: Routledge.

Hui, L., Ng, G. Y. F., Yeung, S. S. M., & Hui-Chan, C. W. Y. (2001). Evaluation of physiological work demands and low back neuromuscular fatigue on nurses working in geriatric wards. *Applied Ergonomics, 32,* 479–483.

Knibbe, J. J., & Friele, R. D. (1996). Prevalence of back pain and characteristics of the physical workload of community nurses. *Ergonomics, 39*(2), 186–198.

Massad, R., Gambin, C., & Duval, L. (2000). The contribution of ergonomics to the prevention of musculoskeletal lesions among ambulance technicians. *Proceedings of the IEA2000/HFES 2000 Congress* (4, 201–204). The Human Factors and Ergonomics Society, Santa Monica, California. Nelson, A. (1996). [Risk Analysis of High Risk Patient Handling Tasks in SCI and Nursing Home]. Unpublished raw data from study conducted 1995–1996. Tampa, FL: James A. Haley VA Hospital.

Nelson, A. L., & Fragala, G. (2004). Equipment for safe patient handling and movement. In W. Charney, & A. Hudson (Eds.), *Back injury among healthcare workers* (pp. 121–135). Washington, DC: Lewis Publishers.

Nelson, A. L., Lloyd, J., Menzel, N., & Gross, C. (2003). Preventing nursing back injuries: redesigning patient handling tasks. *AAOHN Journal, 51,* 126–134.

Nelson, A. L., Powell-Cope, G., Gavin-Dreschnack, D., Quigley, P., Bulat, T., Baptiste, A., Applegarth, S., & Friedman, Y. (2004). Technology to promote safe mobility in elderly. *Nursing Clinics of North America, 39*(3), 649–671.

Owen, B. (1987). The need for application of ergonomic principles in nursing. In *Trends in ergonomics: Human factors IV* (pp. 831–838). North Holland: Elsevier.

Owen, B. (2000). Preventing injuries using an ergonomic approach. *AORN Journal, 72*(6), 1031–1036.

Owen, B. D., & Garg, A. (1990). Assistive devices for use with patient handling tasks. In B. Das (Ed.), *Advances in industrial ergonomics and safety*. Philadelphia, PA: Taylor & Frances.

Owen, B., Garg, A., & Jensen, R. C. (1992). Four methods for identification of most back-stressing tasks performed by nursing assistants in nursing homes. *International Journal of Industrial Ergonomics, 9,* 213–220.

Owen, B. D., & Staehler, K. (2003). Approaches to decreasing back stress in homecare. *Home Healthcare Nursing Manual, 21*(3), 180–186.

Schibye, B., & Skotte, J. (2000). The mechanical loads on the low back during different patient handling tasks. *Proceedings of the IEA2000/HFES 2000 Congress* (p. 785). The Human Factors and Ergonomics Society, Santa Monica, California.

Skarplik, C. (1988). Patient handling in the community. *Nursing, 3*(30), 13–16.

Smedley, J., Egger, P., Cooper, C., & Coggon, D. (1995). Manual handling activities and risk of low back pain in nurses. *Occupational and Environmental Medicine, 52,* 160–165.

Wicker, P. (2000). Manual handling in the perioperative environment. *British Journal of Perioperative Nursing, 10*(5), 255–259.

PART II

Best Practices

Evidence-Based Guidelines for Patient Assessment, Care Planning, and Caregiving Practices in Safe Patient Handling and Movement

Audrey L. Nelson

Much of nursing practice is based on tradition, rather than scientific evidence. This leads to unnecessary variation in practice, diminishing quality of care (Institute of Medicine, 2004). The purpose of this chapter is to outline (1) an evidence-based protocol for patient assessment related to patient handling and (2) algorithms to standardize decisions about the type of equipment needed and the number of caregivers needed to perform the task safely. The algorithms are divided into two areas—practices for high-risk patient handling tasks in the general patient population as well as for the bariatric (morbidly obese patient). Evidence is constantly evolving and the algorithms are reviewed and modified annually;

"The views expressed in this article are those of the authors and do not necessarily represent the view of the Department of Veterans Affairs. No claim made to U.S. government material. Contact Author: Audrey.Nelson@med.va.gov."

updates can be found on the Tampa VA Patient Safety Research Center website (www.patientsafetycenter.com) on the "Safe Patient Handling and Movement" page as part of the "Patient Care Ergonomics Resource Guide" or as a separate document "Algorithms for Safe Patient Handling and Movement."

DEVELOPMENT AND VALIDATION OF THE ASSESSMENT TOOL AND ALGORITHMS

A Technical Advisory Group (TAG), working in collaboration with the VHA Public Health and Environmental Hazards, Patient Safety Center of Inquiry (Tampa, FL), and Healthcare Analysis and Information Group, was formed. The TAG developed the assessment tool and an algorithm for each of the key transfer and repositioning tasks. The algorithms were designed to caregivers in selecting the safest equipment and techniques based on specific patient characteristics. These guidelines were originally prepared based on scientific and professional information available in March 2001. These algorithms were tested in three hospitals across the USA, targeting six clinical practice areas (Intensive Care Units; Acute Care Units; Nursing Home Care Units; Outpatient Areas and Clinics, and Emergency Rooms; Operating and Recovery Rooms; and Spinal Cord Injury Units and Rehabilitation Units). The tools were reviewed and approved for use by Veterans Health Administration (VHA) nurse executives, and were subject to external peer review nationally. These tools were published in 2003, in the *American Journal of Nursing* (Nelson et al., 2003). The tools were modified again in 2004 and 2005 based on new evidence related to special conditions likely to affect safe performance of patient handling tasks. Once again, external peer review was used to validate the tool. Users of this guideline should periodically review this material to ensure that the advice herein is consistent with current reasonable clinical practice. As with any guideline, this content provides general direction; professional judgment is needed to assure safety of patients and caregivers.

PURPOSE OF PATIENT ASSESSMENT CRITERIA AND CARE PLAN

Patient assessment criteria can assist caregivers in evaluating critical patient characteristics likely to affect decisions for selecting the safest equipment and techniques for patient handling and movement tasks.

Direct caregivers have become accustomed to manual lifting or using whatever limited lifting aids are available, rather than carefully matching equipment to specific patient characteristics. It is expected that careful use of this assessment and planning tool will improve safety for both patients and caregivers. Patients will receive assistance appropriate for their functional level, assuring safety and comfort, and maximizing their functional capacity. For caregivers, the goals are to decrease the incidence, severity, and costs associated with job-related injuries, as well as decreasing the intensity, duration, and frequency of job-related musculoskeletal pain and discomfort experienced by caregivers performing patient handling tasks. Figure 5.1 depicts an assessment form that can be used in patient care areas for assessing patients including a care plan that can be used to foster unit-based communication.

KEY ASSESSMENT CRITERIA

Key assessment criteria, most likely to affect safe performance of patient handling tasks include:

- Ability of the patient to provide assistance.
- Ability of the patient to bear weight.
- Upper extremity strength of the patient.
- Ability of the patient to cooperate and follow instructions.
- Patient height and weight.
- Special circumstances likely to affect transfer or repositioning tasks, such as abdominal wounds, contractures, or presence of tubes, etc.
- Specific physician orders or physical therapy recommendations that relate to transferring or repositioning patients (e.g., a patient with a knee or hip replacement may need a specific order or recommendation to maintain the correct angle of hip or knee flexion during transfer).

CARE PLAN CONSIDERATIONS

The care plan was designed to communicate decisions about safe patient handling practices among the full array of staff likely to perform these tasks, including across shifts. Decisions focus on (1) the type of task to be completed, e.g., transferring, repositioning, ambulating, or toileting; (2) type of equipment or assistive devices needed; (3) number

Assessment Criteria and Care Plan for Safe Patient Handling and Movement

I.   **Patient's Level of Assistance:**
      _____ Independent— Patient performs task safely, with or without staff assistance, with or without assistive devices.
      _____ Partial Assist—Patient requires no more help than stand-by, cueing, or coaxing, or caregiver is required to lift no more than 35 lbs. of a patient's weight.
      _____ Dependent—Patient requires nurse to lift more than 35 lbs. of the patient's weight, or is unpredictable in the amount of assistance offered. In this case assistive devices should be used.

An assessment should be made prior to each task if the patient has varying level of ability to assist due to medical reasons, fatigue, medications, etc. When in doubt, assume the patient cannot assist with the transfer/repositioning.

II.   **Weight Bearing Capability**   III. **Bi-Lateral Upper Extremity Strength**
      _____ Full   _____ Yes
      _____ Partial   _____ No
      _____ None

IV.   **Patient's level of cooperation and comprehension:**
      _____ Cooperative — may need prompting; able to follow simple commands.
      _____ Unpredictable or varies (patient whose behavior changes frequently should be considered as "unpredictable"), not cooperative, or unable to follow simple commands.

V.   **Weight: _____   Height: _____**
      Body Mass Index (BMI) [needed if patient's weight is over 300][1]:_____
        If BMI exceeds 50, institute Bariatric Algorithms

The presence of the following conditions are likely to affect the transfer/repositioning process and should be considered when identifying equipment and technique needed to move the patient.

VI.   **Check applicable conditions likely to affect transfer/repositioning techniques.**
_____ Hip/Knee Replacements   _____ Respiratory/Cardiac Compromise
_____ History of Falls   _____ Wounds Affecting Transfer/Positioning
_____ Paralysis/Paresis   _____ Amputation
_____ Unstable Spine   _____ Urinary/Fecal Stoma
_____ Severe Edema   _____ Contractures/Spasms
_____ Very Fragile Skin   _____ Tubes (IV, Chest, etc.)
_____ Postural Hypotension   _____ Severe Pain/Discomfort
_____ Severe Osteoporosis   _____ Fractures
_____ Splints/Traction

Comments:_____
_____
_____
_____
_____
_____
_____

Algorithm	Task	Equipment/ Assistive Device	# Staff
1	Transfer To and From: Bed to Chair, Chair To Toilet, Chair to Chair, or Car to Chair.		
2	Lateral Transfer To and From: Bed to Stretcher, Trolley.		
3	Transfer To and From: Chair to Stretcher, or Chair to Exam Table.		
4	Reposition in Bed: Side-to-Side, Up in Bed.		
5	Reposition in Chair: Wheelchair and Dependency Chair.		
6	Transfer Patient Up from the Floor		
Bariatric 1	Bariatric Transfer To and From: Bed to Chair, Chair to Toilet, or Chair to Chair		
Bariatric 2	Bariatric Lateral Transfer To and From: Bed to Stretcher or Trolley		
Bariatric 3	Bariatric Reposition in Bed: Side-to-Side, Up in Bed		
Bariatric 4	Bariatric Reposition in Chair: Wheelchair, Chair or Dependency Chair		
Bariatric 5	Patient Handling Tasks Requiring Access to Body Parts (Limb, Abdominal Mass, Gluteal Area)		
Bariatric 6	Bariatric Transporting (Stretcher)		
Bariatric 7	Bariatric Toileting Tasks		

Sling Type: Seated_____ Seated (Amputation)_____ Standing_____

Supine_____ Ambulation_____ Limb Support_____

Sling Size: _____

Signature: _____

Date: _____

[1]If patient's weight is over 300 pounds, the BMI is needed. For Online BMI table and calculator see: http://www.nhlbi.nih.gov/guidelines/obesity/bmi_tbl.htm

FIGURE 5.1   Assessment criteria and care plan for safe patient handling and movement.

of caregivers needed to complete the task safely; and (4) special consid-erations, such as sling type. Baptiste, Matz, Evitt, and McCleerey (in press) have published an article with in-depth information on sling types and applications.

PROCESS FOR USING ASSESSMENT AND PLANNING CRITERIA

The specific process for assessment and care planning may vary by facil-ity, patient population, or level of care. However, key elements need to be considered and integrated into the assessment and care planning pro-cess for safe patient handling and movement.

- Who completes the assessment?
- How often assessment is completed?
- How will the information be commuted to all staff?
- What is the process for updating/revising the plan as needed?

WHAT IS AN ALGORITHM?

An algorithm is a clinical tool based on evidence, useful for making healthcare decisions. The pathway directs the caregiver through a series of questions (diamond boxes) and provides optimal responses for ac-tion—in this case what type of equipment should be used and how many caregivers are needed to perform the task safely. The tool is designed for efficiency, that is, it limits inputs to the most critical decision points in a finite number of steps.

PURPOSE OF ALGORITHMS

Algorithms standardize practice based on the most current evidence, rather than each caregiver relying on their own training and experi-ences to make decisions, which could result in significant variations in the way a patient is transferred during a single hospital stay. Building on the patient assessment criteria, algorithms should be used as guides when planning the following patient high-risk patient handling tasks. As with clinical practice guidelines, they are not prescriptive and should not replace sound clinical judgment.

WHO SHOULD USE THE ALGORITHMS?

These algorithms are targeted for persons directly involved with patient handling and movement, such as registered nurses, licensed practical nurses, nursing assistants, orderlies, physical/occupational therapists, radiology technicians, patient care technicians, and other care providers.

CONTENT OF THE ALGORITHMS

Patient handling tasks were selected based on the level of risk, frequency that the tasks were performed, and the availability of evidence to support practices. Initially, there was some concern that use of patient handling equipment might have a negative affect on the patients' functional status over time. A National Task Force was convened including representatives from the Association of Rehabilitation Nurses (ARN), American Physical Therapy Association (APTA), and the Veterans Administration (VA). A position paper was developed by this group and published (APTA/ARN/VA Task Force on Safe Patient Handling and Movement, 2005). Initially, patient handling tasks focus on the general patient population; however, as the need for specialized care of the bariatric patient emerged, these algorithms were added.

Algorithms for General Patient Population

- Vertical transfers (patient starts and ends in a seated position), such as transfer from bed to chair, chair to toilet, wheelchair to bedside chair, or car to wheelchair (see Figure 5.2).
- Lateral transfers (patient starts and ends lying in a prone or supine position), such as bed to stretcher, bed to prone cart, or bed to bath trolley (see Figure 5.3).
- Combined vertical/lateral transfers (patient moved from seated position to supine position, or vice versa), such as transfer from wheelchair to stretcher or wheelchair to examination table (see Figure 5.4).
- Repositioning in bed, including side to side or moving a patient up toward the head of the bed (see Figure 5.5).
- Repositioning in chair, including pulling a patient who was slumped down in a dependency chair or wheelchair, or repositioning to prevent pressure ulcers (see Figure 5.6).
- Picking a patient up off the floor, post-fall (see Figure 5.7).

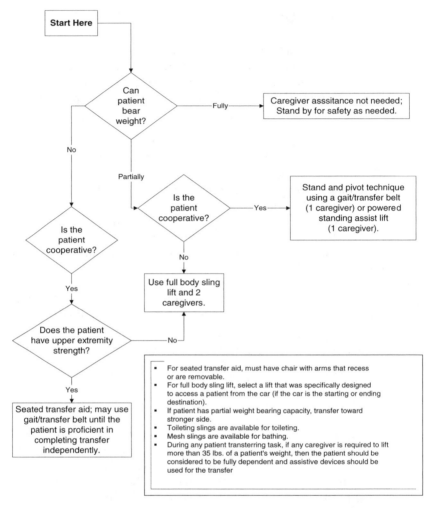

FIGURE 5.2   Algorithm 1: transfer to and from: bed to chair, chair to toilet, chair to chair, or car to chair.

Algorithms for Bariatric Patient Population

- Vertical transfers (patient starts and ends in a seated position), such as transfer from bed to chair, chair to toilet, chair to chair, or car to chair (see Figure 5.8).
- Lateral transfers (patient starts and ends lying in a prone or supine position), such as bed to stretcher or trolley (see Figure 5.9).

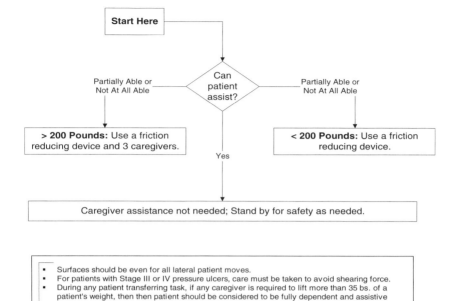

FIGURE 5.3   Algorithm 2: laterial transfer to and from: bed to stretcher, trolley.

- Repositioning in bed, including side to side or moving a patient up toward the head of the bed (see Figure 5.10).
- Repositioning in a chair, wheelchair, or dependency chair (see Figure 5.11).
- Patient handling tasks requiring access to body parts (limb, abdominal mass, gluteal area) (see Figure 5.12).
- Transport via stretcher (see Figure 5.13).
- Toileting task (see Figure 5.14).

PROCESS FOR USING THE ALGORITHMS

These algorithms should be used as guidelines when planning the following patient transfer and repositioning tasks. Prior to using any of the aforementioned algorithms, careful patient assessment is critical to ensure safe patient handling. The patient characteristics differ among these patients and this diversity needs to be addressed carefully before selection of equipment is determined.

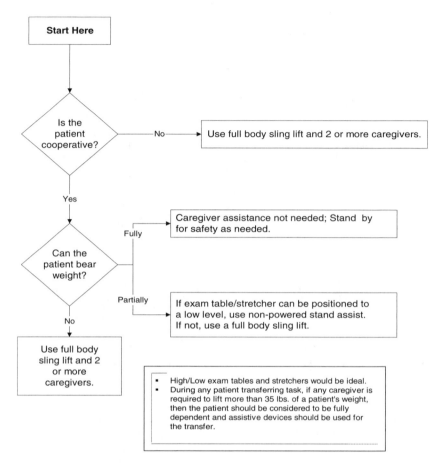

FIGURE 5.4   Algorithm 3: transfer to and from: chair to stretcher, or chair to exam table.

The bariatric patient population poses different challenges in comparison to the general patient population. Some of the associated health problems experienced by the bariatric patient include, but are not limited to: hypertension, respiratory and cardiac disease, diabetes, osteoarthritis, stress incontinence, hyperlipidemia, depression, lack of self esteem, gall bladder disease, and skin breakdown. Distribution of body mass is atypical and affects positioning/posture, turning, entry and egress, medical procedures, hygiene, skin management, breathing, ambulation, and transfers.

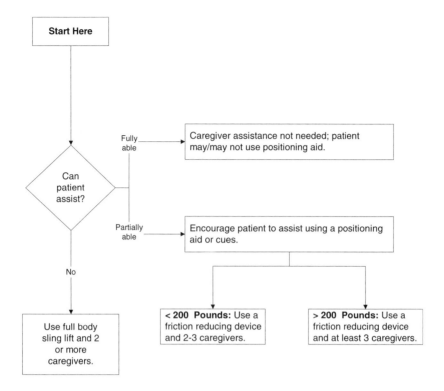

Start Here

Can patient assist?

Fully able → Caregiver assistance not needed; patient may/may not use positioning aid.

Partially able → Encourage patient to assist using a positioning aid or cues.

No → Use full body sling lift and 2 or more caregivers.

< 200 Pounds: Use a friction reducing device and 2-3 caregivers.

> 200 Pounds: Use a friction reducing device and at least 3 caregivers.

- This is not a one person task: DO NOT PULL FROM HEAD OF BED.
- When pulling a patient up in bed, the bed should be flat or in a Trendelenburg position (when tolerated) to aid in gravity, with the side rail down.
- For patients with Stage III or IV pressure ulcers, care should be taken to avoid shearing force.
- The height of the bed should be appropriate for staff safety (at the elbows).
- If the patient can assist when repositioning "up in bed," ask the patient to flex the knees and push on the count of three.
- During any patient handling task, if the caregiver is required to lift more than 35 lbs. of a patient's weight, then the patient should be considered to be fully dependent and assistive devices should be used.

FIGURE 5.5 Algorithm 4: reposition in bed: side to side, up in bed.

Steps in the Assessment Process

1. Patient's functional status
2. Weight-bearing ability
3. Upper extremity strength to safely transfer and ambulate
4. Cooperation and comprehension

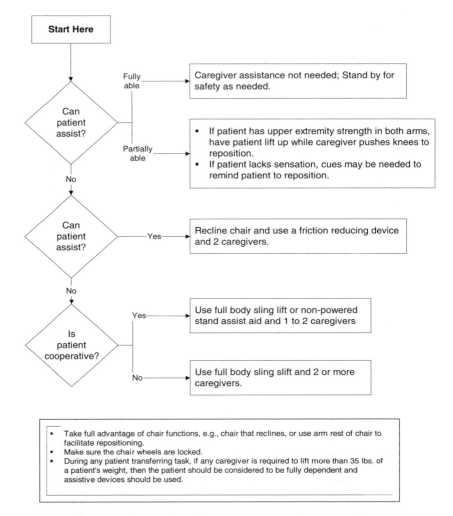

FIGURE 5.6   Algorithm 5: reposition in chair: wheelchair and dependency chair.

5. Height, weight, and body mass index (BMI)
6. Other assessment parameters may include: amputations, contractures/spasms, fractures, hip/knee limitations, skin integrity, a history of falls, paralysis/paresis, postural hypotension, respiratory compromise, severe edema, osteoporosis, fragile skin integrity, and/or pain/discomfort

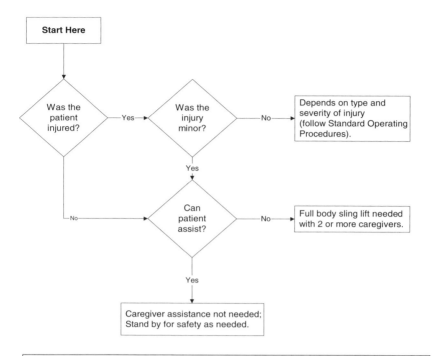

FIGURE 5.7   Algorithm 6: transfer patient up from the floor.

These bariatric algorithms should be used as guides when plan-ning patient transfer and repositioning tasks (Figures 5.8–5.14) if the patients' BMI exceeds 50. These algorithms can be used by many healthcare professionals including registered nurses, licensed practical/vocational nurses, nursing assistants, orderlies, physical/occupational therapists, radiology technicians, patient care technicians, and caregiv-ers in the home.

CASE STUDY

Mr Smith is 55 years old and has been in the critical care unit for 1 week and has to undergo a medical procedure. He was admitted for cardiac

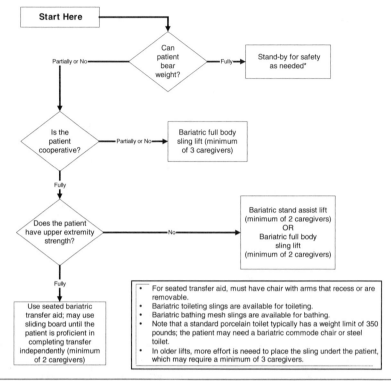

FIGURE 5.8   Bariatric algorithm 1: bariatric transfer to and from: bed/chair, chair/toilet, or chair/chair.

problems and presented with a history of falls, respiratory compromise, and postural hypotension. Although able to comprehend, Mr Smith is unable to cooperate and is required to be in a high-fowlers' position due to respiratory compromise. Mr Smith has a stature of 1.75 m and weighs 273 kg. He needs to be first transferred laterally on to a stretcher, and then transported from his room in critical care to X-ray, which is located on another floor.

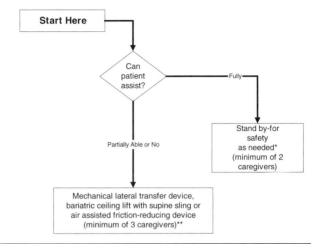

- The destination surface should be about 1/2" lower for all lateral patient moves.
- Avoid shearing force.
- Make sure bed is the right width, so excessive reaching by caregiver is not required.
- Lateral transfers should not be used with speciality beds that interfere with the transfer. In this case, use a bariatric ceiling lift with supine sling.
- Ensure bed or stretcher doesn't move with the weight of the patient transferring.
- ** Use a bariatric stretcher or trolley if patient exceeds weight capacity of traditional equipment.

* "Stand-by for safety." In most cases, if a bariatric patient is about to fall, there is very little that the caregiver can do to prevent the fall. The caregiver should be prepared to move any items out of the way that could cause injury, try to protect the patient's head from striking any objects or the floor and seek assistance as needed once the person has fallen.
* Assure equipment used meets weight requirements. Standard equipment is generally limited to 250-350 lbs. Facilities should apply a sticker to all bariatric equipment with "EC"(for expanded capability) and a space for the manufacturer's rated weight capability for that particular equipment model.
- If patient has partial weight-bearing capability, transfer toward stronger side.
- Consider using an abdominal binder if the patient's abdomen impairs a patient handling task.
- Identify a leader when performing tasks with multiple caregivers. This will assure that the task is synchronized for increased safety of the healthcare provider and the patient.
- During any patient transferring task, if any caregiver is required to lift more than 35 lbs of a patient's weight, then the patient should be considered to be fully dependent and assistive devices should be used for the transfer.

FIGURE 5.9   Bariatric algorithm 2: bariatric lateral transfer to and from: bed/stretcher, troller.

Steps in the Process of Using Bariatric Algorithms

1. Patient's functional status: dependent
2. Weight-bearing ability: partial
3. Upper extremity strength to safely transfer and ambulate: none
4. Cooperation and comprehension: not cooperative, but can understand instructions

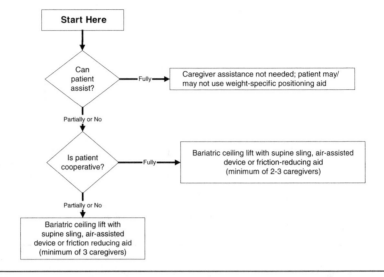

- When pulling a patient up in bed, place the bed flat or in a Trendelenburg position (if tolerated and not medically contraindicated) to aid in gravity; the side rail should be down.
- Avoid shearing force.
- Adjust the height of the bed to elbow height.
- Mobilize the patient as early as possible to avoid weakness resulting from bed rest. This will promote patient independence and reduce the number of high risk tasks caregivers will provide.
- Consider leaving a friction-reducing device covered with drawsheet, under patient at all times to minimize risk to staff during transfers as long as it doesn't negate the pressure relief qualities of the mattress/overlay.
- Use a sealed, high-density, foam wedge to firmly reposition patient on side. Skid-resistant texture materials vary and come in set shapes and cut-your-own rolls. Examples include:
  - Dycem (TM)
  - Scoot-Guard (TM): antimicrobial; clean with soap and water, air dry.
  - Posey-Grip (TM): Posey Grip does not hold when wet. Washable, reusable, air dry.

- If patient has partial weight-bearing capability, transfer toward stronger side.
- Consider using an abdominal binder if the patient's abdomen impairs a patient handling task.
- Assure equipment used meets weight requirements. Standard equipment is generally limited to 250-350 lbs. Facilities should apply a sticker to all bariatric equipment with "EC"(for expanded capabity) and a space for the manufacturer's rated weight capability for that particular equipment model.
- Identify a leader when performing tasks with multiple caregivers. This will assure that the task is synchronized for increased safety of the healthcare provider and the patient.
- During any patient transferring task, if any caregiver is required to lift more than 35 lbs of a patient's weight, then the patient should be considered to be fully dependent and assistive devices should be used for the transfer.

FIGURE 5.10 Bariatric algorithm 3: bariatric reposition in bed: side to side, up in bed.

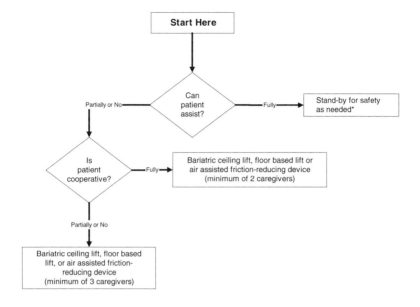

FIGURE 5.11   Bariatric algorithm 4: bariatric reposition in chair: wheelchair, chair, or dependency chair.

5. Height, weight, and BMI:
   • Height = 1.75 m, weight = 273 kg, BMI = weight/(ht²)−
     BMI= 89
6. Medical conditions of concern during transport: postural hypotension, respiratory, and cardiac compromise
   • BMI is over 50; therefore, institute bariatric algorithm #2 for
     lateral transfer and #6 for patient transport

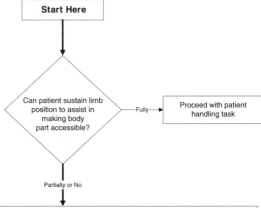

FIGURE 5.12 Bariatric algorithm 5: patient handling tasks requiring access to body parts (limb, abdominal mass, gluteal area).

Decision Process (Lateral Transfer From Bed to Powered Stretcher)

1. Can Mr Smith assist? No, fully dependent
2. Options are to use a mechanical lateral transfer device, a bariatric ceiling lift with supine sling or air-assisted device with minimum of three caregivers. Certain checks should be performed prior to moving Mr Smith:
   - Check that the weight capacity of the stretcher can accommodate 273 kg prior to moving Mr Smith
   - Ensure that the wheels are securely locked so that bed or stretcher does not move during lateral transfer

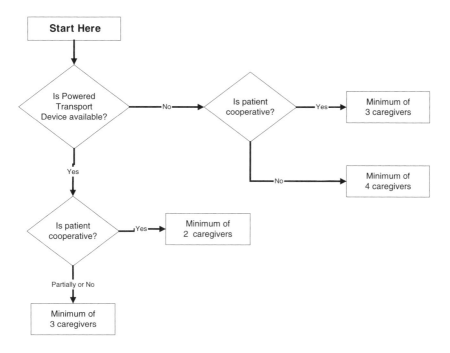

FIGURE 5.13   Bariatric algorithm 6: bariatric transporting (stretcher).

- If bed has an air mattress, it should be fully inflated so that the surface is firm before the transfer begins
- Make sure stretcher is the right width for Mr Smith

Decision Process (Transport of a Bariatric Patient)

1. Is powered transport device available? Yes
2. Is Mr Smith cooperative? No
3. Use a powered stretcher and a minimum of three caregivers

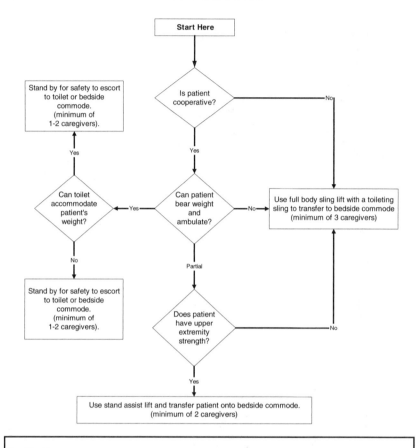

FIGURE 5.14 Bariatric algorithm 7: toileting tasks for the bariatric patient.

- Certain checks should be performed prior to moving Mr Smith
- Ensure stretcher has the capability of maintaining high-fowler's position
- Secure Mr Smith in the stretcher

REFERENCES

Baptiste, A., Matz, M., Evitt, C., & McCleerey, M. (in press). Evaluation of sling use in patient safety. *Rehabilitation Nursing*.

Institute of Medicine (IOM). Committee on the Work Environment for Nurses and Patient Safety (including Nelson, A. L.). (2004). *Keeping patients safe*: *Transforming the work environment of nurses*. Washington, DC: National Academic Press.

Nelson, A., Owen, B., Lloyd, J. D., Fragala, G., Matz, M. W., Amato, M., Bowers, J., Moss-Cureton, S., Ramsey, G., Lentz, K. (2003). Safe patient handling and movement. *American Journal of Nursing, 103*, 32–43.

APTA/ARN/VA Task Force on Safe Patient Handling and Movement. (2005). Position paper: safe patient handling and movement tasks in rehabilitation settings. *PT Magazine of Physical Therapy April 2005*, 48–52.

Physical therapists and other health care providers sustain work-related musculoskeletal injuries as a result of patient handling and movement. A national task force, with representation from the American Physical Therapy Association, the Association of Rehabilitation Nurses, and the Veterans Health Administration, has developed a white paper and issued a list of six recommendations to enhance patient and provider safety during patient handling and movement.

Strategies to Improve Patient and Health Care Provider Safety in Patient Handling and Movement Tasks

A Collaborative Effort of the American Physical Therapy Association, Association of Rehabilitation Nurses, and Veterans Health Administration

Introduction

Over the past few decades, there has been growing concern over the increasing number and severity of musculoskeletal injuries associated with patient handling tasks, especially in nursing personnel. This concern has led to reports recommending patient handling technologies be used in place of traditional manual lifting.

These recommendations have triggered debate between physical therapists (PTs) and rehabilitation nurses (RNs). On one hand, with the nursing shortage and high rates of injuries among nursing personnel, the recommendations are viewed as a necessary safety measure. On the other hand, over use of mechanical lifting devices could affect patient functional status and independence. This paradox has triggered debate and has hindered efforts to promote safe patient handling and movement in rehabilitation settings.

In order to address these concerns, the Veterans Health Administration (VHA) convened a National Task Force, consisting of representatives from the Association of Rehabilitation Nurses (ARN), American Physical Therapy Association (APTA), and the VHA. The purpose of this task force was to develop a position paper, balancing the needs of all three organizations into a workable solution. Our goal was to find a way to effectively incorporate the most recent evidence on safe patient handling and movement into rehabilitation settings.

Purpose

The purpose of this white paper is to promote collaboration between rehabilitation nurses and physical therapists to address the mutual goals of improving:

1. Safety of patients during handling and movement tasks.
2. Functional status and independence of patients to achieve optimal rehabilitation potential.
3. Safety of care providers during patient handling and movement tasks.
4. Utilization of evidenced based research on safe patient handling and movement.
5. Communication between interdisciplinary team members regarding safe patient handling methods.

Recommendations

After careful consideration of current practice and research, APTA, ARN, and the VHA Task Force on Safe Patient Handling and Movement make the following recommendations in order of priority:

1. Implement the OSHA Ergonomics for the Prevention of Musculoskeletal Disorders: Guidelines for Nursing Homes.

a. Establish an interdisciplinary team responsible for reviewing and implementing the OSHA guidelines.
b. Utilize or adapt algorithms in the guidelines for making decisions about safe patient movement.
c. Establish organizational policies and procedures based on the guidelines.

Discussion: In 2003, the Occupational Safety and Health Administration (OSHA) promulgated voluntary guidelines for nursing homes for the prevention of musculoskeletal injuries. Though this document was written to assist in reducing the number and severity of work-related musculoskeletal injuries in nursing homes, they have application to many clinical settings, including rehabilitation. The guideline recommendations were based on current scientific evidence, and existing practices and programs, and were reviewed by various professional and trade associations, labor organizations, and other stakeholders. The guidelines address a process for protecting workers and recommendations for identification of problems and implementation of solutions for patient lifting and repositioning.

2. Build and support a culture of safety in rehabilitation settings that protects staff as well as patients.

Discussion: There is a difference in the culture of the two disciplines in regards to occupational safety. Professional level educational programs for physical therapists emphasize self-protection and patient safety during all patient handling and movement tasks. This results in the development of a culture of safety that transcends into practice. In contrast, professional level educational programs in nursing emphasize patient safety but lack emphasis in self-protection. This results in a culture where self-protection is not valued. For the last 30 years, nurses have appeared on the Occupational Safety and Health Administration's (OSHA) top 10 list of professions with work related injuries.3 A reduction in occupational injuries associated with patient handling can only occur when the nursing profession and nurses themselves recognize this risk and take steps to promote their own safety. This will require a paradigm shift for the nursing profession and a change in the way nurses are taught in schools of nursing. Recognition that the culture of self-sacrifice contributes to the risk of injury in nursing is a necessary first step in the paradigm shift to accept self-preservation and safety as high priorities. With the shortage of RNs, health care organizations need every nurse to be injury free.

3. Improve communication channels between nurses and physical therapists to facilitate safe patient handling and movement tasks.

    a. Collaborate on patient handling policies.
    b. Develop process for initial plans of patient care with on-going updates.
    c. Develop routine interdepartmental meetings to discuss staffing and equipment needs.

Discussion: The development of a facility-wide policy that outlines patient handling and movement tasks should be the product of collaboration among nursing, physical therapy, and other rehabilitation professional staff and address issues such as bed mobility, transfers, ambulation and gait, wheelchair activities, and other activities of daily living. This policy should include provisions for discussing current patient level of cooperation, bed mobility assistance needs, transfer level, wheelchair level, ambulation and gait level, special equipment needs, and functional goals. Status should be updated at pre-set intervals to account for fluctuation in endurance and/or mentation. The policy should also outline the availability, storage location, function, and maintenance of all equipment. Finally, it should create a common language for all personnel to minimize error in decision-making, interpretation of patient care plans, and status evaluation. This policy may be further modified to meet special needs of individual patient care units.

The periodic review of staffing allocation and equipment needs are recommended to appropriately respond to an ever-changing patient population. While the appropriate selection of assistive and patient handling equipment can minimize the physical effort of personnel, these equipment still require one or more staff for safe operation, and the allocation of staff should continually meet the demands of the patient population. Interdepartmental meetings give staff the opportunity to request input on use or function of equipment; problems with equipment use, storage, and maintenance; and may generate ideas for improved staff utilization.

4. Develop policies and procedures for the therapeutic use of patient handling equipment.

  a. Select equipment that first provides safety for staff and patients.
  b. Select equipment with features that, as appropriate, allow for or promote active use of the assistive equipment by the patient for some therapeutic benefit.

Discussion: Selection of patient handling equipment should assure the safety of providers and patients yet not jeopardize the patient's rehabilitation potential. Various patient handling equipment may be used as assistive devices during rehabilitation, thereby increasing the patient's familiarity and independence with the device while decreasing the risk for developing occupational musculoskeletal injuries in staff. Institutional policy and procedures should include the following objectives so to prevent injury and maintain optimum rehabilitation potential:

- Train all staff in the proper and safe operation of all equipment.
- Use valid and reliable algorithms and patient assessment tools. (An example is included in the OSHA Guidelines.)
- Encourage patient participation in the use of assistive equipment (eg some sit/stand lifts can be used as an ambulation aid).
- Conduct an individualized functional assessment of each patient to assure techniques for assistance with movement are appropriate.
- Provide consistency in the use of equipment by both physical therapy and nursing staff.

5. Develop competency-based assessments that demonstrate proficiency for use of all patient handling equipment used on the respective patient care unit, including return demonstration.

Discussion: All new physical therapy and nursing staff should be introduced to patient handling equipment used by the facility during orientation. Once the employee has been assigned to a specific patient care unit, additional training should be provided to include the use, function, maintenance, and proper storage of the equipment. Adequate hands-on practice with the equipment must be provided and include the operation from provider and receiver roles, and coaching on how to train patients and family members on the appropriate use of the equipment. Employees should be required to demonstrate competency through active methods such as role playing and teaching other staff members (otherwise known as return demonstration).

A system for ongoing assessment of competency with these devices should be incorporated into existing channels for behavioral observation and professional development. In this way, there is a simple expansion of a familiar and accepted process rather than a new method that requires extensive introduction, orientation, and teaching. For example, proper use of equipment could be added to a checklist used by safety or ergonomics teams that perform random or periodic walkthroughs, an existing peer-review process, or an existing system for positive reinforcement whenever good practices are observed. More importantly, the continual review process helps to integrate appropriate use of equipment into the safe patient handling culture.

6. Encourage research that supports the improvement of patient and staff safety while maximizing patient rehabilitation potential.

   a. Investigate the cost-effectiveness of ergonomics interventions.
   b. Investigate the impact of injury-risk reduction to physical therapists.
   c. Determine the efficacy of patient handling equipment when integrated into therapeutic activities.

Discussion: To enhance administrative support and resource allocation for purchasing appropriate patient handling equipment, cost effectiveness studies are needed to build a solid business case for safe patient handling interventions. Consideration of the direct and indirect costs associated with workplace injuries must be addressed and may include assessment of the costs of medical care, absenteeism, replacement, rehiring, training, work restrictions, insurance and worker's compensation premiums, productivity, quality of care, and the impact on morale.

While the integration of safe patient handing practices that emphasizes the use of assistive equipment has been encouraged in nursing personnel, little is documented about the impact of injury reduction strategies when these devices are integrated into physical therapy practice. Further research is needed to investigate the effect of patient handling and movement on physical therapy staff injury rates, the use of equipment as a means to assist in reaching rehabilitation goals while preventing injury, and the attitudinal changes required to incorporate safe patient handling techniques using equipment into physical therapy practice.

REFERENCES

1. Panel on Musculoskeletal Disorders and the Workplace; Commission on Behavioral and Social Sciences and Education; National Research Council; and Institute of Medicine. 2001.

2. US Department of Labor, Occupational Safety and Health Administration. *Ergonomic Guidelines for Nursing Homes*. 2002. Available at www.osha.gov/ergonomics/guidelines/nursinghomes/final_nh_guidelines.html. Accessed February 24, 2004.

3. US Department of Labor, Occupational Safety and Health Administration. Table SO1. Highest incident rates of total nonfatal occupational injury and illness cases, private industry, 2001. Accessed October 31, 2003. Available at www.bls.gov/iif/oshwc/osh/os/ostb1109.pdf.

ADDITIONAL RESOURCES

Bernard, BP. Musculoskeletal disorders and workplace factors. U.S. Department of Health and Human Services; 1997.

Bohannon RW. Horizontal transfers between adjacent surfaces: forces required using different methods. *Archives of Physical Medicine and Rehabilitation*. 1999;80: 851–853.

Bork BE, Cook TM, Rosecrance JC, Engelhardt KA, Thomason ME, & Wauford IJ. Work-related musculoskeletal disorders among physical therapists. *Phys Ther*. 1996;76(8):827–835.

Buss IC, Halfens RJG, & Abu-Saad HH. The most effective time interval for repositioning subjects at risk of pressure sore development: a literature review. *Rehabilitation Nursing*. 2002:27(2), 59–66.

Caboor DE, Verlinden MO, Zinzen E, Van Roy P, Van Riel MP, & Clarys JP. Implications of an adjustable bed height during standard nursing tasks on spinal motion, perceived exertion, and muscular activity. *Ergonomics*, 43(10), 1771–1780.

Cohen-Mansfield J, Culpepper II WJ, & Carter P. Nursing staff back injuries: prevalence and costs in long term care facilities. *AAOHN Journal*. 1996: 44(1), 9–17.

Collins, JW, & Owen BD. (1996). NIOSH research initiatives to prevent back injuries to nursing assistants, aids, and orderlies in nursing homes. *American Journal of Industrial Medicine*. 1996:29:421–424.

Cromie JE, Robertson VJ, & Best MO (2000) Work-related musculoskeletal disorders in physical therapists: Prevalence, severity, risks and responses. *Phys Ther*. 2000:80(4):336–351

Daynard D, Yassi A, Cooper JE, Tate R, Norman R, & Wells R. Biomechanical analysis of peak and cumulative spinal loads during simulated patient-handling activities: a substudy of a randomized controlled trial to prevent lift and transfer injury of health care workers. *Applied Ergonomics*, 2001:32:199–214.

Dybel, GJ. Ergonomic evaluation of work as a home health care aide. Unpublished doctoral dissertation, University of Massachusetts Lowell. 2000.

Estryn-Behar M, Kaminski M, Peigne E, Maillard MF, Pelletier A, Berthier C, Delaporte MF, Paoli MC, & Leroux, JM. Strenuous working conditions and musculo-skeletal disorders among female hospital workers. *International Archives of Occupational and Environmental Health*. 1990:62(1):47–57.

Granata KP, & Marras WS. Relation between spinal load factors and the high-risk probability of occupational low-back disorder. *Ergonomics*. 1999:42(9):1187–1199.

Hignett S. Ergonomic evaluation of electric mobile hoists. *British Journal of Occupational Therapy*. 1998:61(11): 509–516.

Hignett S. Work-related back pain in nurses. *Journal of Advanced Nursing*. 1996:23:1238–1246.

Hignett S, Crumpton E, Ruszala S, Alexander P, Fray M, and Fletcher B. *Evidence-Based Patient Handling: Tasks, Equipment and Interventions*. New York: Routledge; 2003.

Lagerstrom M, Hansson T, & Hagberg M. Work-related low-back problems in nursing. *Scandinavian Journal Work Environment Health*. 1998:24(6): 449–464.

Marras WS, Davis, KG, Kirking BC, & Bertsche PK. A comprehensive analysis of low-back disorder risk and spinal loading during the transferring and repositioning of patients using different techniques. *Ergonomics*. 1999:42(7):904–926.

Myers D, Silverstein B, & Nelson NA. Predictors of shoulder and back injuries in nursing home workers: a prospective study. *American Journal of Industrial Medicine*. 2002:41:466–476.

Ronald LA, Yassi A, Spiegel J, Tate RB, Tait D, & Mozel MR. Effectiveness of installing overhead ceiling lifts: reducing musculoskeletal injuries in an extended care hospital unit. *AAOHN Journal*. 2002:50(3):120–127.

Silverstein B, Viikari-Juntura E, & Kalat J. Use of a prevention index to identify industries at high risk for work-related musculoskeletal disorders of the neck, back, and upper extremity in Washington State, 1990-1998. *American Journal of Industrial Medicine.* 2002:41:149–169.

Ulin SS, Chaffin DB, Patellos CL, Blitz SG, Emerick CA, Lundy F, & Misher L. A biomechanical analysis of methods used for transferring totally dependent patients. *SCI Nursing.* 1997:14(1):19–26.

Winkelmolen GHM, Landeweerd JA, & Drost MR. An evaluation of patient lifting techniques. *Ergonomics.* 1994: 37(5):921–932.

Yassi A, Cooper JE, Tate RB, Gerlach S, Muir M, Trottier J, & Massey K. A randomized control trial to prevent patient lift and transfer injuries of health care workers. *Spine.* 2001:26(16):1739–1746.

Yassi A, Khokhar J, Tate R, Cooper J, Snow C, & Vallentyne S. The epidemiology of back injuries at a large Canadian tertiary care hospital: implications for prevention. *Occupational Medicine.* 1995:45(4):215–220.

US. Department of Labor, Occupational Safety and Health Administration. Table SO1. Highest Incident rates of total nonfatal occupational injury and illness cases, private industry, 2001. Available at www.Bls.Gov/iif/oshwc/osh/os/ostb1109.pdf. Accessed October 31, 2003.

Task Force Participants

Audrey Nelson, PhD RN FAAN
Director Patient Safety Center
Director, HSR&D REAP Patient
Safety
James A Haley VA Hospital
Tampa, FL

Catherine A Tracey, MS, RN
Administrator of Nursing
Havenwood-Heritage Heights
Concord, NH

Marian L Baxter MS MA RN CRRN
Clinical Nurse Specialist
McGuire VA Medical Center
Richmond, VA

Paul Nathenson, MPA BSN RN CRRN
Vice President of Patient Care
Madonna Rehabilitation Hospital
Lincoln, NE

Mary Rosario, BSN RN ANCC
Rehabilitation Staff Nurse
Tampa General Hospital
Tampa, FL

Kathleen Rockefeller, PT ScD MPH MS
Clinical Assistant Professor
Department of Physical Therapy
University of Illinois at Chicago
Chicago, IL

Miriam Joffe, PT, MS, CPE
Sr Consulting Ergonomist
Auburn Engineers, Inc
Austin, TX

Kenneth J Harwood, PT PhD CIE
Director, Practice Department
American Physical Therapy
Association
Alexandria, VA

Kevan Whipple, PT DPT STS CEAS
Senior Staff Physical Therapist
VA Salt Lake City Health Care
System

CHAPTER SIX

Patient Handling Technologies

John D. Lloyd

The healthcare industry recognizes the high risk of injury involved in the manually lifting and transferring of physically dependent patients. The principal element of many patient handling tasks involves either a vertical or horizontal transfer. Vertical patient handling activities include transfer from bed to chair, bed to commode, and chair to commode. Horizontal or lateral patient handling activities include bed to stretcher transfers and repositioning tasks.

Technological solutions are needed to address the prevalence of musculoskeletal injuries in nursing related to patient handling and movement tasks. The purpose of this chapter is to identify, describe, and discuss technologies that make the workplace safer for caregivers performing patient handling tasks. Key technologies are grouped according to principal function. Technologies to assist with vertical transfer of patients include powered full-body sling lifts, floor-based lifts, ceiling-mounted patient lifts, powered standing lifts, non-powered standing aids and gait/transfer belts. Technologies to assist with lateral transfer and repositioning of patients include air-assisted systems, friction-reducing

"The views expressed in this article are those of the author and do not necessarily represent the view of the Department of Veterans Affairs. No claim made to U.S. government material. Contact Author: John.Lloyd2@med.va.gov."

devices, mechanical lateral transfer aids, sliding boards, and transfer chairs. Other new and emerging technologies, which stand to positively impact the nursing profession, such as powered transport devices, are also presented.

TECHNOLOGIES TO ASSIST WITH VERTICAL TRANSFER OF PATIENTS

Powered Full-Body Sling Lifts

Perhaps the most commonly used patient lifting technology is a powered full-body sling lift. A vast number of models and configurations are available and are typically used with patients who have physical and/or cognitive impairments. These lifting devices can be used for almost any type of lift transfer. Powered lifting devices offer many benefits over mechanical or manual alternatives, since caregivers do not have to physically lift or reposition patients. The patient transfer is accomplished with the powered advantage of the patient lift, so there is less risk of injury to the caregiver.

There is a wide variation in the types of slings available for full-body lifts. Newer sling designs are much easier to install beneath patients or residents. When using full-body sling lifts, patients need to be fitted with slings of the right size to ensure that no skin shearing or pressure points exist during the transfer. Emerging patient lift systems are exploring opportunities to integrate the sling into hospital bedding or the patient's clothing, after the innovation proposed by Lloyd and Wilkinson (1999). Alternative new technologies for vertical transfer of patients propose sling-less patient handling, which poses enormous time- and energy-saving potential while affording appropriate considerations to patient safety.

The majority of powered full-body sling lifts are mounted on a portable base; however, use of ceiling-mounted patient lifts is growing dramatically. The portable base and the ceiling-mounted devices have differing advantages. With a ceiling-mounted device, there is no need to maneuver over floors and around furniture; however, transfers are limited to areas where overhead tracks have been installed. Where overhead tracks are not available or practical, portable base lifts can be used.

Floor-Based Lifts

As the category title suggests, floor-based lifts are constructed on a base that is maneuverable across the floor (Figure 6.1). Research by Nelson, Lloyd, Gross, and Menzel (2003) indicates that biomechanical stressors

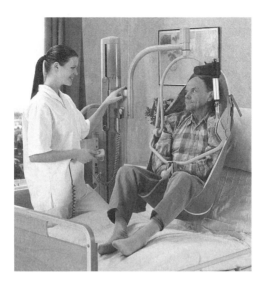

FIGURE 6.1   Floor-based lift with power positioning (courtesy of Arjo USA, Inc.)

imposed on a caregiver are significantly higher during the operation of floor-based lifts versus ceiling-mounted lifts. Further, floor-based patient lifts can be difficult to operate in confined or crowded spaces, such as patient rooms and bathrooms; may be unavailable or inaccessible, especially during high-demand times of the day; necessitate frequent maintenance; and require valuable storage space when not in use. Nevertheless, these common lifting systems continue to play a vital role in safe patient handling and movement.

A new innovation in the market of powered full-body sling lifts is "powered positioning." Typically, while transferring a patient between a supine and a seated posture, the caregiver manually directs the patient's position. This can be achieved by exerting a physical force against straps located on the sling, or using a positioning handle designed into the hanger bar. These forces can impose a biomechanical stress on the wrist, elbow, and shoulder joints of the caregiver in direct proportion to the weight of the patient. Powered positioning affords the nurse the facility to change a patient's posture using the powered advantage of the patient lift system. This new technology is available for both floor-based and ceiling-mounted patient lifts.

It is imperative that the motor of the powered lift is compatible with patients' weight, therefore lift capacities have increased considerably over the past decade. The present standard of 270 kg (600 lb) for most floor-based and ceiling lift systems affords facility-wide coverage that should adequately address the needs of all by the most overweight patients. Lifts are now available with expanded capacity for morbidly obese patients up to 1000 pounds.

Ceiling-Mounted Patient Lifts

Ceiling-mounted lifts are becoming a favorable investment in many hospitals across North America and Europe. These lifts differ from floor-based lifts in that they are suspended from tracks mounted overhead and therefore do not impose on limited floor space, nor do they require storage.

The two principal ceiling lift configurations are single-track and transverse track. A single-track system follows a dedicated path, therefore, patient care activities involving vertical transfers are limited to this specific path. A transverse coverage system has a boom mounted perpendicular to two end tracks, thereby affording considerably broader coverage within the room (Figure 6.2).

Ceiling-mounted patient lifts can be used safely for patients who are at times combative, unpredictable, or have cognitive deficits. There is no need to maneuver over floors or around furniture; therefore, unlike the floor-based lifts, ceiling lifts can accomplish patient transfers safely in tight spaces with fewer caregivers.

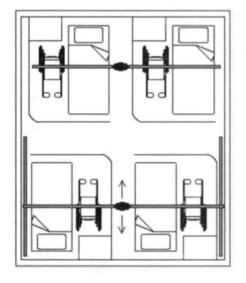

Single track coverage

Transverse track

FIGURE 6.2   Single Track vs. Transverse Coverage for Ceiling Lift Systems

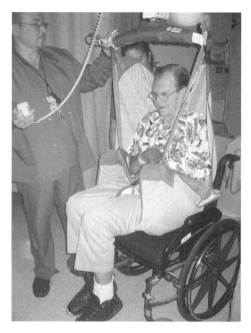

FIGURE 6.3 Ceiling-Mounted Patient Lift
(Note the caregiver does not need to work around the base of the lift, increasing safety for both the nurse and the patient)

These devices have a few drawbacks, including geographical restrictions of the lift based on where tracks are installed. Further, a ceiling lift system might represent a greater capital investment on the part of the healthcare facility, since more systems would be required. However, this added cost may be offset by increased productivity of staff who do not have to search and wait for available floor lifts, as well as increased longevity of these systems due to reduced daily operation of the technology (Figure 6.3).

Powered Standing Lifts

Powered standing lifts provide an alternative to full-body sling lifts and are particularly useful for patients who are cognitively coherent, partially dependent, and have some weight-bearing capabilities. These lifts are excellent for moving patients in and out of chairs and for toileting tasks. Powered standing assist lifts have a relatively small base and are therefore easily maneuvered in restricted areas,

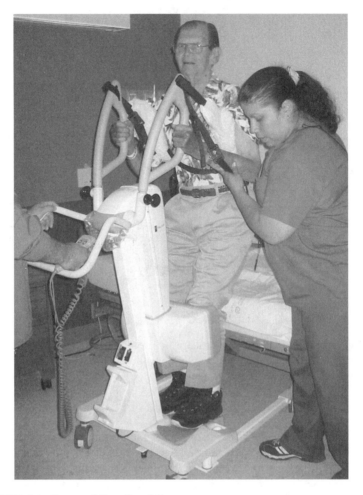

FIGURE 6.4 Powered Standing Lift

such as small bathrooms. There are some variations in the sling design, but the basic concept is of simple design, and it is very easy to place around the patient's torso. This type of sling allows unrestricted access to the patient's lower body for the purpose of toileting (Figure 6.4). Powered standing lifts should not be used with patients who are at times combative, unpredictable, or have cognitive deficits. Further, the equipment is not suited for patients with limited weight-bearing capability.

Non-Powered Standing Aids

Some patients or residents who have reduced leg and/or abdominal strength, such as elderly or post-surgical patients, may need only a little support to stand. In this case, they can help themselves if they have a support to grasp. Various types of devices can be provided to assist a patient in transferring from a seated to a standing position by allowing them to hold on to a secure device and pull themselves up. These devices may be freestanding or attached to beds. The device illustrated in Figure 6.5 may be operated with or without the assistance of a caregiver.

Hospital bed rails are often used by patients to help them stand. However, bed rails are considered restraints if used to prevent the individual from getting out of bed, and because they pose an entrapment risk, the routine use of bed rails is being discouraged (Hoffman, Powell-Cope, Rathvon, & Bero, 2003). Some manufacturers offer standing and repositioning aids as alternatives to traditional rails (see Figure 6.6).

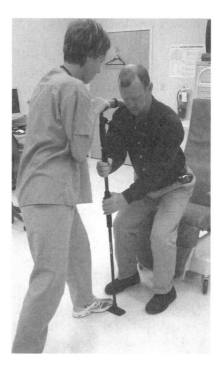

FIGURE 6.5   Non-Powered Standing Aid

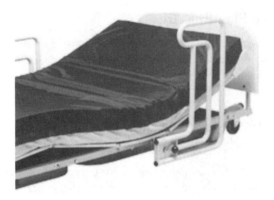

FIGURE 6.6 Bed with Side-Assist Rail

Gait/Transfer Belts

An object with handles is often easier to grasp. This concept is applied to patient handling in the form of gait/transfer belts, which patients can wear around their waist. The belt itself can provide appropriate coupling, or additional straps may be sewn into the belt. These belts provide convenient handles for the caregiver(s) to grasp when assisting the transfer of a partially dependent patient, as shown in Figure 6.7. Small hand-held slings that go around the patient can also facilitate a transfer by providing handles.

Gait/transfer belts are a low-cost transfer solution suitable for patients who have weight-bearing capability and require only minimal assistance. These options should not be used with patients who are at times combative, unpredictable, or have cognitive deficits. Further, the belts are not useful for bariatric patients.

TECHNOLOGIES TO ASSIST WITH LATERAL TRANSFER OF PATIENTS

One of the highest risk tasks in nursing is transferring a patient between the bed and the stretcher. This type of transfer involves the caregiver reaching over the stretcher to the bed, and then physically pulling the patient across to the stretcher. This task forces the caregiver into an awkward posture, likely to cause musculoskeletal discomfort and possible cumulative injury. The use of lateral transfer aids can correct poor postures by reducing reach and pulling, thus reducing the risk of

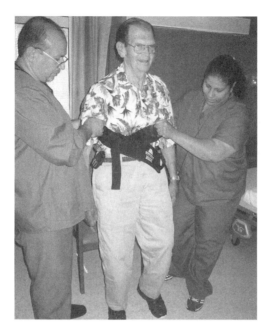

FIGURE 6.7   Gait/Transfer Belt

injury to the caregivers. Several different types of laterals transfer aids are commercially available: (a) air-assisted systems; (b) friction-reducing devices; and (c) mechanical lateral transfer aids.

Air-Assisted Lateral Transfer Systems

Air-assisted lateral transfer systems are an interesting innovation for patient handling tasks, similar in concept to a hovercraft. A deflated specialty air mattress is installed beneath a dependent patient, onto which a portable air supply is attached that inflates the mattress (see Figure 6.8). Air flows through perforations in the underside of the mattress, the upthrust of which helps to overcome the weight of the patient, thereby reducing the forces required to execute a lateral transfer. In fact, Lloyd and Baptiste (in press) determined that air-assisted devices may be up to 85% efficient, meaning that forces equal to only 15% of the patient's mass are required to perform the transfer. Even with the use of an air-assisted lateral transfer device, two caregivers are needed to perform this task safely for patients up to 100 kg; for heavier patients, three or more caregivers may be required.

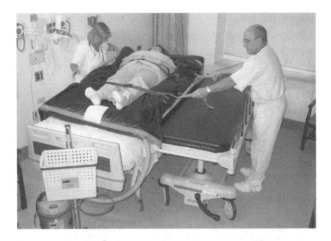

FIGURE 6.8   Air-Assisted Lateral Transfer System (courtesy of AirPal, Inc.)

Air-assisted transfer systems are appropriate when performing lateral transfers or repositioning tasks involving patients who can offer caregivers limited or no assistance. These technologies are particularly suitable for patients with special medical conditions, such as pressure sores or burns. Air-assisted lateral transfer systems have no maximum weight capacity and therefore may be appropriate for use with bariatric populations, provided that sufficient staff are available to assist in the transfer.

Friction-Reducing Devices

As the name suggests, these devices, often constructed of smooth synthetic fabrics, offer friction-reducing properties to facilitate the lateral transfer or repositioning of patients that can offer limited or no assistance. Friction-reducing devices effectively reduce the forces required to execute the transfer, minimizing biomechanical loading on the caregiver's arms and back. Properly designed handles and pull straps can improve the caregivers' grasp and reduce forward reach during transfers, as shown in Figure 6.9, which improves caregiver's posture.

The device is positioned beneath the patient similar to a transfer board, providing a smoother surface on which to slide the patient more easily. To perform the task safely, the two transfer surfaces should be at the same height, preferably at elbow level of the caregivers. Similar to the recommendation for air-assisted lateral transfer systems, for patients up to 100 kg, two caregivers are needed to safely transfer a patient using a friction-reducing device; for heavier patients, three or more caregivers are required.

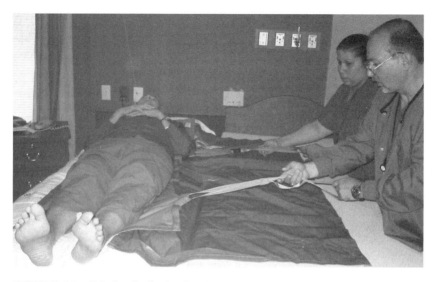

FIGURE 6.9   Friction Reducing Device
(note the long handles which minimize the dangerous need to reach across the surface to complete the task)

Several friction-reducing devices are commercially available, each offering subtle differences in design, which may be used for the lateral transfer or repositioning of dependent patients. If the task needs to be performed frequently, it is advantageous to store this low-cost device at the bedside for ready access. Such devices should be provided in sufficient number, and training in their correct use is imperative to successful implementation.

The weight capacity of these devices is between 100 and 150 kg, depending on the manufacturer. Friction-reducing device are therefore not suitable for the horizontal transfer or repositioning of bariatric patients. For patients with pressure ulcers, care must be taken to avoid shearing force when inserting the device as well as when moving across surfaces.

Mechanical Lateral Transfer Aids

Mechanical lateral aids are those devices that provide mechanized or powered assistance for patient horizontal transfers and therefore eliminate the need to manually slide patients, thus substantially reducing the risk of injury to caregivers. Stretchers are available that are height adjustable and have a mechanical means of transferring a patient on and

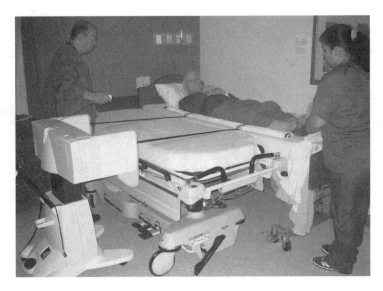

FIGURE 6.10   Mechanical Lateral Transfer Aid

off the stretcher. Mechanical means of mechanizing the lateral transfer are also available as independent options able to be used alongside most beds and stretchers, as illustrated in Figure 6.10.

Mechanical lateral transfer aids are highly recommended when handling bariatric populations (morbidly obese patients), due to the higher range of weight capacities. The mechanical features of these products make them more costly than air-assisted aids and friction-reducing devices; however, the benefits of purchasing these devices far outweigh the cost.

Sliding Boards

Sliding boards are usually made of a smooth rigid material with a low coefficient of friction. The lower coefficient of friction allows for an easier sliding process. These boards act as a supporting bridge when slide transfers are performed. Some manual assistance may still be required to move the patient; however, sliding boards do offer considerable improvement at a minimal cost. The illustrated example is suitable for independent or assisted transfers between wheelchair and bed (see Figure 6.11).

This device maximizes the patient's functional level, promoting patient independence. Sliding boards are most appropriate for patients with limited to no weight-bearing capability that have strong upper body strength, such as a person with paraplegia. The patient may need

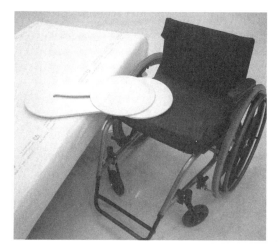

FIGURE 6.11 Sliding Board

limited caregiver assistance or may be able to perform the task independently. Sliding boards should not be used for patients who cannot offer
any physical assistance, obese patients, or patients who have cognitive
deficits and/or difficulty following instructions.

Transfer Chairs

Some new wheelchairs and dependency chairs can be converted into
stretchers where the back of the chair pulls down and the leg supports
come up to form a flat stretcher. These devices facilitate the horizontal transfer of patients between the chair and the bed or stretcher,
thereby eliminating the need to perform a vertical transfer (see
Figure 6.12).

NEW AND EMERGING TECHNOLOGIES

Equipment to Facilitate Patient Transport

Transporting a patient in a bed, stretcher or wheelchair requires significant effort, particularly over uneven terrain, carpeting, or long distances.
This task typically requires two or more staff to perform safely. Powered transport devices have recently been introduced into the market of
patient handling technologies to address this problem. These devices can
be attached to the head of the bed or stretcher and are motorized, thereby

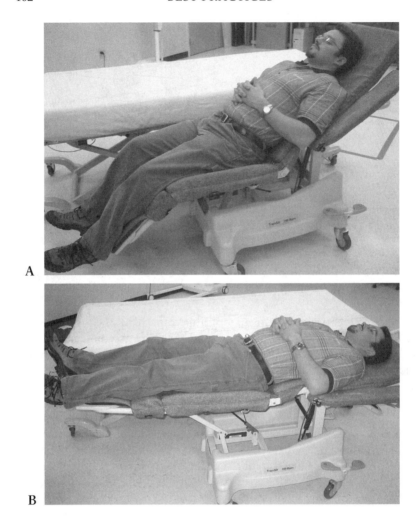

FIGURE 6.12   Transfer Chair

assisting in variable-speed propulsion of the patient (see Figure 6.13). This low-cost device can be used for patient transport throughout a hospital or nursing home, requiring only one caregiver to perform the task. Some newer higher end stretchers and hospital beds have integrated motorized capability. Although more convenient and able to eliminate storage problems, which is otherwise an issue for the independent transport devices, the integrated systems can be considerably more expensive and serve only one patient at a time.

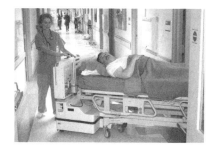

FIGURE 6.13 Powered Bed Mover (courtesy of Dane Industries, Inc.)

FUTURE DIRECTIONS

One particular identified need that still requires an adequate solution involves the egress of dependent patients from private vehicles. A suitable device should minimize caregiver's awkward postures and manual lifting of patients. This technology should be able to adjust to cars and trucks of any height and accommodate patients of any weight. Such a technology would be of tremendous benefit, particularly for caregivers working in hospital emergency departments.

Substantial progress has been made over the past decade in the development of patient transfer equipment. Patient handling technologies are now prevalently available to meet the needs of nearly all patient populations. Collaborative efforts between healthcare organizations, staff, and manufacturers have resulted in considerable product improvements. These collaborative efforts hold great promise for the creation of a safer environment for nursing staff as well as for a positive impact on the quality of patient care.

REFERENCES

Hoffman, S., Powell-Cope, G., Rathvon, L., & Bero, K. (2003). BedSAFE: evaluating a program of bed safety alternatives for frail elders. *Journal of Gerontological Nursing, 29*(11), 34–42.

Lloyd, J., & Wilkinson, S. (1999). Integrated sling for patient lift manipulation. Department of Veteran's Affairs Patents and Licensing office.

Nelson, A., Lloyd, J., Gross, C., & Menzel, N. (2003). Preventing nursing back injuries. *AAOHN Journal, 51*(3), 126–134.

CHAPTER SEVEN

After-Action Reviews

Mary Matz

Frontline employees amass a wealth of information regarding their jobs and work environment. This knowledge is invaluable in building a safe workplace and building a culture of safety. The use of After Action Review (AAR) functions to tap this knowledge, allowing for improvement in workplace safety and empowering staff with responsibility for their own safety.

AAR is a highly successful method of transferring knowledge that is used in high-performing organizations, such as the United States Army. It is a method for transferring knowledge that a team has learned from doing a task in one setting, to the next time the same task is performed in a different setting (Dixon, 2000). This process moves unique knowledge that an individual holds into a group setting so that the knowledge can be integrated, understood by the whole team, and used when individuals face similar circumstances. The Veteran's Health Administration (VHA) describes AAR as a way for a whole clinical team to learn from the experiences of one staff member (Veterans' Health Administration Patient Safety Center, 2002). Often, knowledge generated in work settings is not shared and therefore is not usable by others. AAR offers a way to effectively share safe methods for completing patient handling tasks, as well as

"The views expressed in this chapter are those of the author and do not necessarily represent the vew of the Department of Veterans Affairs. No claim made to U.S. government material. Contact Author: Mary.Matz@med.va.gov."

a way to share and learn from near misses and injuries. AARs provide a structured method for making tacit knowledge explicit among team members, thus usable next time a team member faces a similar task. An AAR functions as a vehicle to *share* information between co-workers in order to decrease the risk of a reoccurrence of an injury/incident or a near miss. Additionally, use of the AAR process embeds organizational knowledge transfer and improvement into an organization's work culture.

This chapter highlights the application of AAR to decrease injuries from patient handling activities. It also relays information on the characteristics and structure of AARs in general, and specifically as used in the Army and VHA. Additionally, guidelines for use of the VHA process and training suggestions are given. But first, the relationship of AAR to knowledge transfer and ultimately an effective culture of safety will be explored.

AAR AS A MECHANISM OF KNOWLEDGE TRANSFER

The ultimate goal of this text and other safety improvement initiatives is to create an effective culture of safety in which staff can be confident that their workplace is physically safe and where management and staff work together for the safety of all. In such a safety culture, employees accept responsibility for their own safety as well as the safety of their co-workers.

What is Knowledge Management and Knowledge Transfer?

Certainly, a requirement for an effective culture of safety is to have control measures that decrease risk from hazards in the work environment, such as patient handling equipment, but support structures must also be in place. Knowledge management and knowledge transfer are such integral support structures. There is no single definition (Shin, Holden, & Schmidt, 2001) or definitive procedure accepted by all (Pffefer & Sutton, 2000), but the goal of knowledge management is to ensure that needed knowledge is made available by fostering the sharing of information. When such knowledge is shared, it benefits organizational performance (O'Dell & Grayson, 1998). Knowledge transfer is defined by Dixon (2000) as the sharing of common knowledge, what we learn in our work. He says common knowledge can either be tacit (residing in people's heads) or explicit (written down into a series of steps or guidelines). For our purposes, knowledge transfer is considered to be the transmission of information intended to effect actions taken in response to hazardous conditions/circumstances in the healthcare work environment, thus decreasing risk of injury.

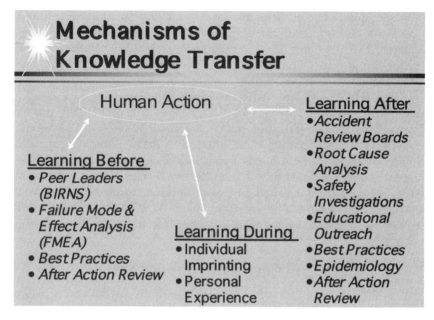

FIGURE 7.1 Mechanisms of knowledge transfer (Powell-Cope & Matz, 2002).

Mechanisms of Knowledge Transfer

There are three mechanisms of knowledge transfer related to human actions and safety-related occurrences: "learning before," "learning during," and "learning after" (see Figure 7.1). Unfortunately, most knowledge regarding workplace safety is transferred after the fact, after an incident has occurred. The topic of this chapter, AAR, provides a mechanism for "learning after" as well as "learning before."

AAR BACKGROUND

The US Army uses AAR to improve its performance and readiness, develop leaders, and evolve its safety culture doctrine. Although acceptance and diffusion was at first slow, it is now institutionalized and a standard Army procedure. Not only does AAR apply to training exercises, field units, and field activities, but high-ranking Army officials also utilize this knowledge transfer mechanism (Garvin, 2000).

Organizations outside of the military have also adopted AAR, and with each organization, the process varies in focus, data used, length of meetings, number of participants, level of facilitation, and more (Signet Consulting Group, 2000, Overview: AARs). Organizations that have adopted AARs as a part of their organizational culture include Shell and Harley-Davidson (Darling & Perry, 2000), BP-Amoco, Motorola, and General Electric (Gurteen, 2000).

The VHA inclusion of AAR as a key program element in their research study, *VISN-Wide Deployment of a Back Injury Prevention Program for Nurses: Safe Patient Handling and Movement* (Nelson et al., in review) was successful. Staff participation in the VHA AARs fostered knowledge transfer among staff, which led to increased feelings of value and importance and improved perception of professional status. An evaluation of AARs revealed them as important to the prevention of musculoskeletal injuries because factors surrounding an injury or near miss were discussed to reduce reoccurrence of a similar incident (Nelson et al., in review).

AAR CHARACTERISTICS—GENERAL

Gurteen (2000) describes the use of AAR in organizations as a powerful tool because it can be applied across a wide spectrum of events. A precipitating event can be as small as a short phone call or as large as a major project dealing with a complex issue. He notes though that each "event" typically has a purpose, a start point, an end point, and has measurable objectives. He offers three types of AAR: (1) formal, (2) informal, and (3) personal.

Formal AARs

They involve pre-planning and preparation of supportive materials. They usually take time to conduct, are scheduled beforehand, and are conducted where best supported. Often an external observer/data recorder is present. A formal AAR would be conducted at the end of a major project.

Informal AARs

They require much less or no preparation planning, time, and materials. They can be held spontaneously, with just-in-time training. Anyone can conduct this type of AAR. They are held as needed and held wherever appropriate.

Personal AARs

They are held by an individual to evaluate an action. A personal AAR held with a mentor or coach increases the benefit of such an AAR.

Importantly, lessons learned can be both immediate and personal as well as shared with other interested individuals (Gurteen, 2000).

When shared, knowledge generated in work settings is usable. AAR provides a structured process to facilitate this. Garvin (2000) compares AARs to "chalk talks," where players and coaches gather around a chalkboard after a game to evaluate the team's recent performance. The team and coaches discuss what went right, what went wrong, and how to improve the game the next time. These chalk talks, as AARs, give a framework for knowledge transfer and making learning routine (Garvin, 2000).

Darling and Perry (2000) stress that successful AAR comes about not by simply perfecting the AAR process, but by ensuring AAR fits the organization's culture and goals. Rather than the process itself, management must keep focused on the goal of creating a culture where people naturally ask what was learned from an experience or activity and how can the learning experience be applied to their work (Darling & Perry, 2000).

CHARACTERISTICS

In the Army, AARs are brainstorming sessions held immediately after an important event or activity to review assignments. They identify successes and failures, and recommend performance improvement recommendations. The process can be formal or informal, may be comprised of large or small groups, and may last for minutes to hours to days. On occasion, a series of AARs are needed to deal with a complex situation. Army recommendations include that AARs be comprised of a diverse, democratic group and participants should speak as much as 75% of the time. They are not lectures or debates. There must be honest and even exchange between all involved, superiors and subordinates. And, as Garvin quotes the Army's chief of staff, there must be "recognition that disagreement is not disrespect" (Garvin, 2000 [p. 4]). Importantly, the same four questions are always used to initiate discussion (Garvin, 2000).

1. What did we set out to do?
2. What actually happened?
3. Why did it happen?
4. What are we going to do the next time?

Garvin (2000) emphasizes that for the Army, use of skilled facilitators is critical. Facilitators introduce the topic, keep the group focused, establish and enforce ground rules, monitor and maintain the schedule, facilitate transition from one question to the next, and summarize the resulting action plans. Importantly, they set the tone of the exchange,

hopefully, one of openness and candor and a willingness to set aside traditional lines of authority (Garvin, 2000).

The Army strives for constructive AARs through the use of ground
rules enforced by facilitators. Tact and civility are required, and personal
attacks are prohibited. No negative information is allowed to be relayed
to superiors and impact the person who admits to a mistake or error.
AARs are considered opportunities for learning, not avenues to blemish
personal records (Garvin, 2000).

As noted previously, the AAR was instituted as part of a comprehensive program for decreasing risk from patient handling injuries in a VHA
sponsored research project, *VISN-Wide Deployment of a Back Injury
Prevention Program for Nurses: Safe Patient Handling and Movement*
(Nelson et al., in review). This innovative solution to address nursing
injuries tested a newly developed patient care ergonomics program
designed to create safer working environments for nurses who provide
direct patient care. The program included several key elements that were
phased in over time. The first program element implemented was the unit
peer leader (see Chapter 9) and then AAR followed close behind. The
AAR process was implemented early on to foster openness and increase
awareness for the program. Throughout the program implementation
process, AARs were used to keep a pulse on program activities and staff
concerns.

AAR was included as a program element because it offered an
effective means to learn from both injury incidents as well as near-miss
or close call incidents, ones in which an injury did not occur, but could
have. AARs were held in order to share knowledge about an incident to
prevent its reoccurrence. The AAR process was also used to discuss a
problem situation prior to the occurrence of a near-miss or injury event.
An additional desired benefit of utilizing AAR was that it had the potential to become a part of the workday routine and this maximizes patient
safety. In acknowledging the fact that everyone makes mistakes and creating an openness of discussion surrounding those mistakes, AARs fostered team building and provided a means to implement changes quickly,
thus having a real effect on injury prevention.

Based on Gurteen's (2000) description, an informal AAR process
was used in Nelson's (in review) program. During AARs, the goal was
for staff to feel free to share knowledge without fear of embarrassment
or blame. AARs were most successful when held on a regular basis,
either scheduled at the same time every day or after some defined unit
or work, such as after morning care was completed. Powell-Cope and
Matz (2002) maintained that routine meetings held frequently would be
easier to keep brief and highly focused. And, completing them frequently
allowed staff to become more comfortable with the process and learn

from experience without placing blame. They recommended opening AAR participation to everyone involved in direct patient care on a unit. Participants could include RNs, LPNs, NAs, PTs, OTs, etc. Every person's ideas and perspective were considered necessary for a clear picture of what occurred. And, all needed to have an opportunity to express ideas for improvements. This openness and acceptance fostered a sense of responsibility that resulted in staff buy-in and safety improvements. Guidelines for AAR, as conducted in the VHA, can be found below. Key questions used for the safe patient handling program included (Veterans' Health Administration Patient Safety Center, 2002):

1. What happened?
2. What was supposed to happen?
3. What accounts for the difference?
4. How could the same outcome be avoided the next time?
5. What is the follow-up plan?

RELEVANCE OF AAR QUESTIONS

As in the military, the goal of the VHA questions is to engage participants in open discussion based on objective facts without blaming individuals. The VHA and the Army's first two questions are basically the same but reversed. The intent of these two questions are to clarify the difference between what happened and what was supposed to happen. Certainly, this can be quite difficult. In order to know "what was supposed to happen," clear goals and standards are a must. In a healthcare setting, policy must define the proper and appropriate method for performing patient care activities. The VHA study instituted a No-Lift policy to make certain that expectations were clear. When describing "what actually happened," having more than one participant involved in the incident may result in different accounts of the same incident. The military deals with these circumstances by adopting the majority opinion or view (Garvin, 2000).

The question, "What accounts for the difference?" fills in the gap between what happened and what was supposed to happen. Brainstorming skills are used to generate as many explanations as possible, and problem-solving skills determine which explanations realistically explain the underlying reasons for an incident. During this process, the complete and honest exchange of thoughts and ideas is paramount to success of the AAR.

The last two questions: "How could the same outcome be avoided the next time?" and "What is the follow-up plan?" are used to develop a plan of action. Participants are usually eager to offer solutions, and they flow easily after a situation is well understood. Garvin (2000) noted that the Army recommends focusing on things that participants can fix, rather than on external forces outside of their control. The VHA AAR process not only allows for but also encourages verbalization of any and all recommendations for consideration. It was felt that a free flow of ideas encourages input and fosters creativity.

TIPS FOR SUCCESSFUL IMPLEMENTATION OF AARs

Leadership support of AARs at all levels is important. This facilitates establishment of AAR in the organizational structure. Such organizational support will drive implementation, but middle management and direct care staff "buy-in" and support are also essential to the success of AAR. Management must demonstrate support by allowing time away from patient care for training and participation in AARs, and they must demonstrate leadership skills by taking immediate and appropriate actions based on staff recommendations. If recommendations are made with no follow-up by management then staff will not see the value of participation.

Management must demonstrate trust and support by ensuring the process is a non-punitive one. And, both management and staff must facilitate a climate of openness and candor and ensure AAR trust is not breached. Staff must demonstrate respect for co-workers by allowing all comments and being non-judgmental. They must accept responsibility for their own work environment by taking action and being part of the solution. This can be demonstrated by initiating AARs. Staff must take responsibility for follow-through of AAR recommendations. And, someone must begin the process of opening up and admitting mistakes, setting an example for co-workers. Peer leaders or an AAR champion might begin this process. As well, knowledge and understanding of staff incentives for participating in AAR will increase success.

GUIDELINES FOR USE OF AAR PROCESS ASSOCIATED WITH SAFE PATIENT HANDLING

The following relays information on the format used for the VHA AAR process; then limitations and benefits of healthcare AARs are presented.

AAR BASICS

What is an AAR?

- AAR is basically a brainstorming session using structured questions to gather information.

What Prompts the Use of an AAR?

- AARs should be held for (1) injuries, (2) near-miss incidents, and (3) safety issues that have not resulted in either near-miss incidents or injuries. Although it is easy to identify the need for an AAR when an injury occurs, it might be less so for near-miss incidents and non-incident safety issues. It is very important though to utilize near-miss and non-incident safety issues to proactively address safety concerns. The use of AAR for such enables "learning before" an incident and will prevent injuries from occurring. An additional benefit of conducting such AARs is that these occur more frequently than injuries, increasing the regular use of AAR. VHA, Army, and other organizations stress the importance of the frequency and regularity of scheduled AAR meetings.
- AAR can also be used to identify what went "right." The AAR questions can identify activities where groups and individuals are performing well. Garvin notes that such positive activities are often difficult to recognize, but if their accomplishments are to be repeated, the underlying causes of success need to be identified (Garvin, 2000).

When are AARs Held?

- Meeting times will vary, but they should fit in with the routine of the unit and be held at a convenient time so that as many staff as possible can attend. They can be held immediately after an incident occurs or they can be held as regularly scheduled meetings. For example, a nursing home care unit may hold AARs once a week after shift report is given, while another unit may decide to hold them immediately after every patient or staff safety near miss and injury incident occurs.

How often Should AARs be Held?

- VHA, Army, and other organizations stress the importance of the frequency and regularity of scheduled AAR meetings (Garvin,

2000; VHA Patient Safety Center, 2002). The more often AAR meetings are held, the more routine they become and the more comfortable participants are with the process. This helps to keep meetings short and to the point. Regular use also results in the incorporation of AAR into the culture of an organization and the adoption of the mindset that AAR "completes" an assignment or activity. And, in doing so, it facilitates knowledge transfer as a part of the daily work routine.

Where are AARs Held?

- If possible, hold AARs in the location of the incident or location of the safety issue of concern. When this is not possible, AARs can be conducted in the staff break room or other convenient staff meeting area.

How Long Should an AAR Last?

- AARs are most effective when meetings are brief and to the point. Use of the questions facilitates focus on the problem area of concern, so 15 min is usually ample time for AAR meetings.

Who Should Participate in an AAR?

- The more and varied minds focused on the safety issue, the better the chance that appropriate and successful solutions will come forth. Each participant's information as well as perspective is critical to obtain a complete picture of what happened. As well, the more participants involved, the greater the number who will benefit from the experience and incorporate information learned into future actions. So, involve as many staff members as possible, but because of the priority of patient care, participation is usually limited to less than 10, which is a manageable number for AAR. Good participation will facilitate the group process and feelings of ownership, thus influencing the success of the corrective actions. The focus of the safety issue or injury will drive who actually participates. Certainly, frontline nursing staff should join in, but it may also be appropriate for therapy staff or others to participate. Management does not usually participate. Shift work makes participation more difficult. In order to successfully address this barrier, conduct AARs on the same issue during all shifts.

Who Initiates an AAR?

- All staff members should be empowered to initiate an AAR. AARs are staff-driven rather than management-driven.

Who Should Lead/Facilitate an AAR?

- As noted previously, AARs are staff-driven, so any staff member can take the leadership role. Having said that, it is helpful to have a leader/facilitator with good communication and group process skills, who is respected by his/her co-workers. A good facilitator can also help participants recognize system and process problems that may require managerial action.

What Information is Written Down? What Notes are Taken?

- There are no formal minutes. AARs are conducted in order to provide a mechanism for staff to learn from their experiences and mistakes as well as those of others. Providing a blame-free, open environment is essential to AAR success. For this reason, during the AAR, it is recommended that only informal notation of recommendations occurs. Participants should feel more at ease to openly discuss their ideas and circumstances surrounding an error or near-miss if no official notes are taken and they are comfortable that they are not at risk of blame or punishment. Notes are for follow-up and informational use only. Depending on the wishes of the staff on a particular unit, a brief synopsis of the safety issue and solution/s can be written in order to disseminate the information gleaned from the AAR. This may be done to provide non-participating staff with information to help them avoid similar safety errors and injuries.

CONVENING AN AAR

What Happens During an AAR?

The leader/facilitator asks participants to brainstorm about the issue of concern by answering five structured questions. The questions should be asked in the order given. It is imperative to keep participants focused on answering these questions to generate appropriate solutions and keep the duration of the AAR brief.

1. What happened?
2. What was supposed to happen?

3. What accounts for the difference?
4. How could the same outcome be avoided the next time?
5. What is the follow-up plan?

What if the AAR Starts to Become a Non-Productive Gripe Session?

AARs will become non-productive if participants are allowed to depart from answering the specific AAR questions. To make this less likely, when first initiating AAR use, utilize a strong leader/facilitator to ensure participants adhere to the rules of the AAR process. If an AAR becomes non-productive, redirect the discussion by use of the AAR questions.

AAR ETIQUETTE

As in any sanctioned group discussion, proper manners must be adhered to for a productive session. All participants should be allowed to voice their opinions and offer suggestions when they are adhering to the AAR question format. Comments should be limited in duration though, so that all participants desiring to speak have time. One person speaks at a time and no side conversations should occur. All information should be offered to the whole group. AAR discussions should be based on facts without placing blame. Participants must be sensitive to those admitting to and discussing their errors. There must be respect and trust among participants.

AFTER AN AAR

How do AAR Participants Make Sure the Recommendations from the AAR are Carried Out?

Direct and active staff involvement in solutions to safety issues is paramount in empowering staff to take responsibility for the safety of their workplace, so assigning follow-up responsibility to AAR participants is essential. These persons are also responsible for providing status reports at subsequent AARs if necessary.

Who Should Hear about the Outcome of an AAR?

Recommendations and information from the AAR should be made available to all staff who may benefit from the information.

How do Staff who Missed the AAR Learn of the AAR and Outcome/s?

The AAR recommendations are made available to all staff through e-mail, person-to-person, staff meetings, posting on bulletin boards, or any other method that works for the unit.

MONITORING AARs

What Should be Monitored?

It is important to monitor AAR effectiveness and acceptance.

How can this Monitoring be Accomplished?

Acceptance monitoring can be accomplished by tracking the frequency of injury, near-miss, and non-incident safety issue AARs initiated and completed. And, if staff find it acceptable, staff participation can be tracked. Effectiveness can be monitored by tracking recommendations accomplished as well as effective safety practices implemented as a result of AARs. Tracking the time when AARs are being conducted might also be useful. Staff opinions on AAR can be obtained through use of interviews, surveys, or AARs.

Limitations and Benefits of Healthcare AARs

As with the Amy, in healthcare settings, institution of AAR takes time, leadership, and commitment. In a healthcare environment, because of the requirements of patient care and the necessity for shift work, all staff members are not able to participate in every AAR. Nursing staff often cannot just stop and take time away from patient care to join in an AAR. Consequently, methods of AAR information dispersion are needed. Suggestions include using e-mail messages, posting AAR outcomes in break areas, and discussing outcomes at change of shift or one-on-one. Holding the same AAR on each shift overcomes the shift barrier. Management can support AAR by offering incentives such as a reward for participating in a certain number of AARs.

AAR is compatible with other established mechanisms for learning from incidents and injuries such as Root Cause Analysis and Accident Review Boards. The advantage of AAR is that it can become a part of the day-to-day routine of a workplace. AAR, though, is not meant to replace a formal injury incident reporting process. If an injury occurs, staff must adhere to organizational policy and report as required.

Institution of the AAR process provides many benefits for an organization and its employees. Because the AAR process is informal and fosters a blame-free environment, it fosters a workplace that views mistakes and errors as opportunities to learn from rather than negative occurrences. AAR provides a format for identification of problems and solutions to those problems; consequently, staff are able to directly and quickly effect change in their workplace. AAR facilitates open communication and sharing among co-workers. Working toward a common goal, that of a safer workplace, fosters a sense of camaraderie and team values. Ultimately, it is hoped that in any organization, use of AAR will foster an environment in which workers are guided by a collective and joint belief in the importance of safety, with the shared understanding that every member is responsible for safety and therefore upholds the group's safety norms.

TRAINING IN USE OF AAR

What Kind of Training is Needed?

Staff need minimal training but continual use. And, management needs to be trained as well as staff. Training can be given during in-services or as just-in-time training. Posting and distributing AAR brochures help.

What Should AAR Training Include?

Below you will find suggestions for training. All of this material can be offered, or simply a primer on benefits and use of the AAR questions may be sufficient.

Knowledge Transfer. It is suggested to start off with a discussion of the importance and impact of knowledge transfer, in that everyone has information of importance to share. Discuss the fact that staff know most solutions to patient handling safety concerns. As well, relay the benefit of greater numbers and varieties of perspectives on safety issues. And, an explanation of why knowledge transfer mechanisms such as AAR are needed to help decrease risk of injury in patient care environments is important. Also include the importance of and the rationale behind the use of the specific, ordered questions.

Culture of Safety. Tying knowledge transfer and AAR to fostering a culture of safety can also have an impact. Emphasis should be placed on the theory that incidents are most often results of organizational system and process breakdowns rather than individual error or fault. This helps the understanding of the intent of AAR, to not place blame, but to find solutions to the problems and conditions that resulted in an injury, near-miss, or safety issue. It is also important to discuss how working as a team will facilitate not only AAR success but decreased risk of injury.

Guidelines for the Use of AAR Process Associated with Safe Patient Handling. Information found under the section, *Guidelines for Use of the VHA AAR Process Associated with Safe Patient Handling,* should be included: AAR Basics, Holding an AAR, After an AAR, How to ensure AAR success, Monitoring AARs for Acceptance and Effectiveness, Management and Staff Support, and Limitations and Benefits.

Case Scenario. As part of AAR training, be sure to go through a case scenario such as the one that follows. Conducting a practice AAR is also helpful.

Are There Any Training Materials Available?

A printable AAR brochure and an AAR PowerPoint presentation can be found at the VHA website, www.patientsafetycenter.com, under "Safe Patient Handling."

CASE SCENARIO

The following case study can be used in training staff in the AAR process. After each scene, questions are suggested to stimulate group discussion and analyze key points of the case study.

Scene 1

- A nurse manager of a long-term care unit decides to implement AAR after she notices an increase in musculoskeletal injuries among the nursing staff. After the nurse manager explains the process to the staff, they decide to schedule meetings on Monday, Wednesday, and Friday at 11:00 am. This time was selected because most of the morning care is completed by 11:00 and it is before the busy time of care around lunchtime. They also thought that AARs after morning care would help them prevent injuries likely to occur during morning care, a high-risk time for injury because of the lifting, moving and turning of patients that is required for bathing, getting patients out of bed, and feeding.

- *Point of discussion:* For musculoskeletal injury prevention, what might be other good times to conduct AARs? How might the times vary with respect to the type of unit, skill mix of staff, and other considerations? What makes these good times?

Scene 2

- The following day patient care staff assemble after morning care and a facilitator asks "*What happened* during morning care related to staff injuries that everyone could learn from?"
- Sue, an LPN, begins. "I had to get Mr. Walker up because he was lying in a wet bed. You know the problem we have had with his skin. I was late with my meds and I was late getting to the mandatory training class. I *know* I was supposed to use the patient lift to get him up, but I could not find the sling, so I just got him up myself. While I was lifting him I was thinking I am not supposed to be doing this. I guess I was lucky I did not hurt myself."
- *What Happened? Sue manually lifted Mr. Walker out of bed.*
- *Point of discussion:* What other information might be useful in gaining a systems perspective on the problem?

Scene 3

- The facilitator then asks, "*What should have happened* in this situation?"
- Sue responds, "I know I should have looked around for the sling and used the lift, but I was in such a hurry."
- Nancy concurs, "It is so frustrating to have all of these new ceiling lifts but not having the slings where you need them, when you need them. I know I have had trouble finding slings, too."
- Others discuss their experiences related to the lifts and slings. They agree that they "like using the lifts, but that finding slings is a problem."
- *What should have happened? Sue should have found a sling and used the ceiling lift to get a dependent patient such as Mr. Walker out of bed.*

- *Point of discussion:* Was Nancy's comment supportive? How else could you imagine staff responding to Sue's observation?

Scene 4

- Facilitator, "What accounts for the difference?"
- Ron begins, "Well. . . . I might have taken Mr. Walker's sling to use for Mrs. Thomas when I got her up. I could not find *her* sling. I must have forgotten to put it back in the room."
- Nancy responds: "I know that I have looked for slings in patient rooms and could not find them too. If we had a place in every room where everyone knows where to find the sling, that would help!"
- Sue adds, "But, we also do not have enough slings available when some are in the laundry."
- After more discussion, the group decides that the problems of "in accessible slings" is caused by no good location for sling storage in patient rooms and an inadequate supply of slings.
- *What accounts for the difference? Sue could not find a sling for use with the ceiling lift.*
- *Point of discussion:* Why is Ron likely to "confess" his mistake? What do you think Nancy's response to him would be/should be?

Scene 5

- The facilitator asks, "*How can the same outcome be avoided the next time*? How can the problem of inaccessible slings be fixed?"
- Ron suggests: "If there was a hook on the back of every door, we could put the slings there and we would always know where to find them."
- The charge nurse, Rose, replies, "That's a great idea Ron. If we have a place to put the slings in every room, and more of them, we should always be able to find a sling."
- *How can the same outcome be avoided he next time? Ensure slings are available and accessible by installing a sling hook on the back of every patient room door and purchase more slings.*
- *Point of discussion:* What are some other ideas? Do you sense that the culture on this unit is one of learning from mistakes? Why?

Scene 6

- The facilitator asks, "What is the follow-up plan?"
- Charge Nurse: I will put in a work order to have hooks installed on all of the doors."
- Sue says, "In the meantime, I will order more slings for the unit."
- Nancy replies, "Those are good ideas. Sue, if you order 10 slings I will make sure everyone gets the message about where to put them."
- Ron offers, "And I will see to it that the process gets into the unit orientation packet for new employees."
- Sue says: "At next month's AAR meeting I will poll everyone to find out if all staff got the message and if anyone is still having the problem with missing slings."
- Facilitator: "Thanks for another successful AAR!"
- *What is the follow-up plan? Several staff members will complete activities to ensure slings are accessible and follow-up will occur at the next AAR meeting.*
- *Point of discussion:* How likely is it that these changes will be put into effect? Could the charge nurse do anything else to ensure implementation of these actions?

REFERENCES

Darling, M., & Perry, C. (2000). *From post-mortem to living practice: An in-depth study of the evolution of the after action review, executive summary.* Retrieved April 20, 2005, from http://www.signetconsulting.com/downloads/aar_execsummary.pdf

Dixon, N. (2000). *Common knowledge: How companies thrive by sharing what they know.* Boston: Harvard Business School Press.

Garvin, D. A. (2000). The U.S. Army's After Action Reviews: seizing the chance to learn. In *Learning in action, a guide to putting the learning organization to work* (pp. 106–116). Boston: Harvard Business School Press.

Gurteen, D. (2000). Introduction to After Action Review. Retrieved July 19, 2004 from The Gurteen Knowledge Website @ http://www.gurteen.com/gurteen/gurteen.nsf/0/E380DBA5E0F0CC0E80256836006B18A7/.

Nelson, A., Matz, M., Chen, F., Siddharthan, K., Lloyd, J., & Fragala, G. (in review). Development and Evaluation of a Multifaceted Ergonomics Program To Prevent Injuries Associated with Patient Handling Tasks. *International Journal of Nursing Studies.*

O'Dell, C., & Grayson, C. J. (1998). *If only we know what we know: The transfer of internal knowledge and best practice.* New York: Simon & Schuster.

Pffefer, J., & Sutton, R. I. (2000). *The knowing-doing gap: How smart companies turn knowledge into action.* Boston: Harvard Business Scholl Press.

Powell-Cope, G., & Matz, M. (2002). Presentation: Organizational learning through knowledge transfer. VISN 8 Occupational Safety Program Development & Strategic Planning Meeting. Tampa, FL. August 13, 2002.

Shin, M., Holden, T., & Schmidt, R. A. (2001). From knowledge theory to management practice: toward an integrated approach. *Information Processing and Management, 37*, 33–355.

Veterans' Health Administration Patient Safety Center (2002). *After Action Review* [Brochure]. Powell-Cope, G.: Author. Retrieved April 21, 2005, from http://www.patientsafetycenter.com/AAR_rev081103.pdf

Lift Teams

A Proven Method to Reduce Back Injury in Healthcare Workers

William Charney

THE LIFTING TEAM

CHRISTOPHER HEWITT

Recently in the hospital
and in great pain
from broken bones
after an accident,
I had to be lifted
bed to gurney, gurney to
x-ray table (brutally hard), table to chair.

Each time they sent for the Lifting Team:
Solomon, built like a football-player with
a wide smile, and Merwin, smaller, agile,
a savvy bird. Each time Solomon would say,
(seeing the tenseness of fear on my face),
"Don't worry, you'll be alright."
Indeed, their arms held me in a firm cocoon,
I never felt the slightest pain.

When in death's last delirium.
I shall call on the Lifting Team.
They will arrive at my bedside,
and Solomon will say, "Don't worry you'll be alright.
And they will halt my ghastly nose dive into hell,
and lift me up, up, high up
into the fields of the stars."

BACKGROUND

Manual lifting and transfer activities are the job tasks most frequently associated with back injuries in nursing personnel (Caska, Patnode, & Clickner, 1998; Cohen-Mansfield, Culpepper, & Carter, 1996; Garg, Owen, & Carlson, 1992; McAbee & Wilkinson, 1988; Stobbe & Plummer, 1988). Factors contributing to back injuries during lifting and transfer tasks might be organizational, environmental, or personal. Examples of organizational factors include time pressure to perform the task, lack of available lifting aids, and lack of personnel to assist with the lift. Environmental factors include space restrictions, inconvenient or inaccessible lifting equipment or transfer devices, and poor condition of such devices. The personal factor most often associated with back injury during lifting is history of previous back injury or recurrent back injury (Caska et al., 1998).

Efforts to decrease back injuries related to lifting and transferring activities must target organizational, environmental, and personal factors. One such approach with potential to reduce back injuries during lifting and transfer activities in hospital personnel is the lifting team.

DEFINITION OF LIFT TEAMS

A lifting team has been defined as "two physically fit people, competent in lifting techniques, working together using mechanical equipment to accomplish high-risk patient transfers" (Meittunen, Matzke, McCormack, & Sobczak, 1999, p. 311). It has also been referred to as a "lift team," "patient transfer team," or various combinations of these terms. The typical lift team described in the literature consists of two employees responsible for patient transfers within a medical center. Members of the lifting team have been male or female orderlies (Charney, 1992, 1997), an existing hospital transport team (Charney, 2000), or nursing staff (Caska, 2000; Caska et al., 1998). The lift team members are selected using a variety of screening methods, which have included history (e.g., to determine if previous back injury has occurred), physical examination (e.g., range of motion, musculoskeletal strength), and radiograph of the spine to detect abnormalities.

The team is given training in several areas, including anatomy, body mechanics, and use of mechanical lifting and transfer devices. The lifting team has most often been used on the day shift for transfers scheduled ahead of time and conducted during scheduled rounds, as well as for unscheduled lifts at other times via a pager system for the team. The lift team uses mechanical devices for all patient transfers and lifts, except for emergency situations.

There are other necessary components to lift team programs, which include an administrative policy on lifting, mechanical lifting and transfer devices, support of nurse managers, union endorsement, a culture of safety within the facility, and knowledge of the team's existence.

The goal in the healthcare delivery system is to mechanize patient repositioning and transfers in order to reduce the exposure of compressive forces on the lumbar spine. Other industries have mechanized to great advantage in reducing their injury claim rates. One element in the mechanization process is the lift teams, as they are part of the overall model that mandates the use of mechanical equipment during patient transfers and removes nursing exposure to the manual loads. Lift teams put "risk where it can be controlled" in a small team rather than spread out in large nursing department.

The healthcare industry mechanizes for patient diagnostics and treatment; however, the second part of the equation of mechanization for healthcare worker safety is lagging far behind. The manufacturers of lifting equipment and patient movement technology have done a credible job in providing the industry with technical options to protect healthcare workers. The research and development phase of patient movement technology have produced advanced floor lift designs; ceiling-mounted transfer designs; sit-to-stand models; lifts that remove patients from cars, baths, and showers mechanically; lateral transfer stretchers; bariatric lifts; beds that can reposition patients; and repositioning devices from slip sheets to handles on beds that can position patients; and, despite peer review, science showing an extremely positive cost-benefit and payback within 12–24 months for equipment and other short payback periods for program implementation; however, the healthcare industry has been slow to implement these evidence-based approaches. (ANA, 2001; Charney, 2003a; Nelson & Fragala, 2003; Worthington, 2001).

JUSTIFICATION FOR USE OF LIFT TEAMS

Professionalizing the transfer and lifting of patients in healthcare settings has been a viable model for the past decade as the data in this chapter document. The concept considers the number of variables that create an incident and the number of employees exposed. By reducing the number of employees exposed, controlling the injury variables, especially by mandating mechanization, the lift team method has put into practice sound risk management principles.

Lifting is a Skill Rather Than a Random Task

According to Charney, " . . . lifting patients is considered a specialized skill performed by expert professional patient movers who have been thoroughly trained in the latest techniques, rather than a hazardous random task required by busy nurses" (Charney, 1997, p. 300). Patient transfers and repositions are complex movements due to patient individuality, pain thresholds, room spacing, patient weight, etc. There are over 20 different types of patient transfers and repositioning techniques that must be learned from vertical transfers and lateral transfers; sit-to-stand paradigms; walking of patients; dressing patients, car transfers, toileting patients, bathing patients, turning patients, and rolling patients; and ambulance transfers, all of which have been shown to create excessive compressive forces on the spine. Additionally, there are over 20 different types of mechanical equipment available that one must learn to manipulate, including, but not limited to: vertical lifts, lateral lifts, sit-to-stand lifts, bath lifts, shower devices, ceiling lifts, toilet lifts, and car lifts, all with three or four different types of slings to be used for different patients or type of lifts. All these maneuvers and equipment require a specialized skill set to be performed in a safe manner for both patient and healthcare worker. Then there are even more subsets. Bariatric patients pose another risk management challenge and they need to be handled safely and with dignity (Figure 8.1).

Patients have no handles and a 10-pound load lifted away from the body exerts a force of 100 pounds on the lumbar spine (Charney, Zimmerman, & Walara, 1991). The average age of nurses in the USA is 45 years, and many thousands have had a prior back injury, which increases their potential for an acute injury. Obesity in patients has increased the risk to caregivers who lift manually, and the need for a higher level of training to reach the level of risk of exposure has never been mandated by the healthcare establishments. "Professionalizing" the task reduces all the variables due to the expertise of the professional, and this in turn contributes to the safe movement of patients. Concentrating a skill level in professional lift teams creates a safety factor for the staff previously exposed to random lifting. It guarantees that the lift will be done according to all the safest techniques, standards and the use of equipment, applications of training and awareness of lift principles thereby reducing the variables that create injury potential.

Putting Risk Where it can be Controlled

This is a risk management strategy that considers the mathematics of the number of people exposed and the number of variables that contribute

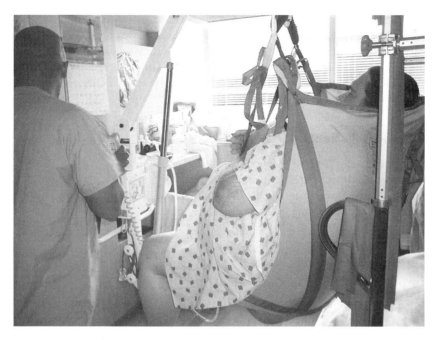

FIGURE 8.1   Lift team working with bariatric patient.

to incidence. In a large nursing department that includes RNs, LPNs, and others exposed to patient transfers, the challenges are formidable that the safety parameters will be followed in ways that reduce biomechanical forces. Training of 1000 employees exposed to patient transfers in an acute care setting, including per-diems and others, on all the parameters of a safe patient handling program is a risk management nightmare given turnover rates of 68% (American Hospital Association (AHA)), vacancy rates of 8.76% (AHA), per-diems, release time for training, etc. The variables are more controllable in a set of teams that the criteria, such as mandated use of mechanical equipment, pre-visualization of lift, and coordination of lift will be followed.

Efficencies in Use of Nursing Staff

The use of lift teams allows the facilities to return injured nurses back to patient bedside care without fear of being exposed to dangerous compressive loads and without fear of reinjury. There are thousands of injured nurses in the USA who are not working due to severe or chronic back pain. This group would be able to return to their careers. Secondly, lift teams allow nurses with previous injuries who are still working, but who are at greater risk for a more acute episode, to work without fear of reinjury. Lift teams are saving nurses an average of 1.5 h per shift, which can be then used for patient bedside care. This time-saving is cost-benefit and patient benefit (Charney, 2003a). Last, lift teams, as a program design, assist in the recruitment of new nurses (Richards, in review) and reduce turnover rates (Hefti et al., 2003).

Enhanced Patient Safety

Lift teams are inherently safer for patients. Lift teams are professional patient transfer experts. In subjective findings (Oregon Health Science University Medical Center), it was found that patients have more confidence in lift teams to move them safely and with less trauma than in staff nurses. Second, there are less patient falls during transfers with lift teams, which reduces hospital liability (Richards, in review).

Improved Quality of Care

Lift teams, due to their training, are able to ambulate complex or totally dependent patients more often, which can amount to shorter patient stay outcomes for this cohort of patients.

TOOLS AND STRATEGIES FOR IMPLEMENTATION

In order to achieve a successful lifting team program, several key components should be addressed. These include selection of lifting team members, training of the lifting team, and lifting team policy components. Each of these areas is outlined further. In addition, a formula for calculating the required number of lifting/transfer devices is provided.

Composition

The facility must determine whether it will use existing or newly hired employees, orderlies, nursing staff, or other job classifications; the number of teams and number of members per team; and the shift(s) to which the team(s) will be assigned.

Selection Criteria

Lifting team members ideally will be free from previous or recurrent back injuries; be physically fit; have normal strength and range of motion; be free from spinal abnormalities that would limit ability to use lifting devices and techniques; work well in teams; be able to assume responsibility; possess good verbal and written communication skills; and be supportive of the program.

Training

Success depends partially on the training of lift team members. The following topics are typically included in job training for lift team members.

- Anatomy and physiology (relevant to preventing back injury)
- Assessment and preparation of patients for transfer
- Assessment of the environment
- Hospital lifting and lift team policies
- Use of mechanical transfer and lifting devices
- Team work
- Communication
- Maintenance of records and logs
- Warm-up and stretching exercises

Training techniques include a combination of classroom lectures, hands-on practice with lifting equipment, return demonstration of team lifts and transfers using mechanical aids and devices, on-site orientation to nursing units where lifts will occur, discussion, and time for questions and answers. The length of the training required for the lifting team may range from 1–2 days to 4–5 days, depending upon whether the lifting team members are new to the facility, their previous experience, size of the facility, type and amount of equipment/devices, etc. In addition to lift team members, other departments and job classifications should receive in-service education regarding the availability and utility of the lifting teams. These include administrators, risk managers, nursing managers, and nursing personnel or other caregivers who will be contacting and utilizing the lifting teams.

Lifting Team Program Policy Components

Typically a facility policy is developed that describes the lift team and encourages nurses to appropriately use the team (e.g., specify whether the team is designed to manage all lifts, all high-risk lifts, all scheduled lifts, etc.), requiring that sufficient equipment is available for the lifts. Further, the policy would clarify the process for how to communicate/activate the lift team (Charney, 1997). Last, the policy can mandate use of lift equipment and describe policy for documentation of activities and requirements for reporting.

IMPLEMENTING PROCESS

Typically implementation begins with the formation of a task force to oversee all aspects of design and implementation. The team includes representation from nursing, patient transportation, administration, safety, therapy, human resources, educators, and other key leaders. It is important to include frontline workers in the development of the team. Key decisions about the operation of the lift team will include the following:

- Types of lifts to be performed
- Units to be covered
- Equipment purchases
- Policy and procedures
- Budgeting and business plan
- Outreach education for facility

Once the team is developed, care must be given to the actual policy and procedures for the facility. Overall these documents need to convey a commitment that is facility-wide. Often the policy/procedures include the following key points and special issues:

1. Nursing must call the team for all total body transfers
2. The patient handling specialist (PHS is defined below) will mediate any problems that arise
3. Creation of a bariatric safety system

Patient lift teams do not support manual lifting. Careful attention needs to be provided for equipment inventory and process for using equipment during patient handling tasks. Special consideration needs to be given in selecting the most appropriate patient handling equipment and slings. It is important to pilot test the new equipment before final purchasing decisions are made.

The next step is to appoint a patient handling specialist (PHS). The person in this key role has leadership responsibilities for daily oversight and problem solving, coordinating patient screening and assessment, and completing reports to lift team task force.

The next decisions focus on screening patients for lifts using a standardized assessment form (Nelson, in press). Patient assessments are typically performed for all new admissions and when the patient's condition changes.

Plans for ongoing administration of the lift team need to be outlined. This includes practical issues such as selection, supervision, training, and scheduling of lift team members, development of documentation of lifts performed, reporting mechanisms, and distribution of teams. Further, a communications system needs to be in place, including on-call systems, hospital rounds, and prioritization of calls.

Lastly a program for monitoring and evaluating the lift team is needed. Data tracking systems should be in place at the onset and performance improvement initiatives implemented over time.

EVIDENCE TO SUPPORT LIFT TEAMS

Lifting teams have been studied for approximately 13 years. The first published study was by Charney (2003b). This study was done at San Francisco General Hospital, a 250-bed acute care facility, and, after 1 year, the rate of injury on the lift team shift was reduced to 0. Since 1997, at least nine other studies by different authors have been published in peer review journals (Caska, 2000; Charney, 1997, 2000; Davis, 1999; Donaldson, 2000; Haiduven, 2003; Hefti et al., 2003; Meittunen et al., 1999). These studies have included approximately 30 different acute care facilities ranging in size from 200 to 1500 beds. There is also additional unpublished data from hospitals showing excellent results. For example, Tampa General Hospital, a 900-bed facility, has been running lift teams for 2 years and in 2004 had only one lost time injury due to patient transfer. In fact all the published studies have shown reductions in lost time injury, lost days, restricted days, compensation and medical dollars; one study (Hefti et al., 2003) also shows reductions in caregiver turnover rates and vacancy rates attributed to the lift teams. A summary of many of these studies can be found in a report by Haiduven (2003) (Figure 8.2).

Additional data from recent case studies are provided in Table 8.1.

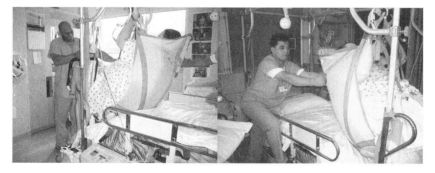

FIGURE 8.2 (Left) Lift team putting patient back to bed. (Right) Lift team positioning bariatric patient.

TABLE 8.1 Case Studies Supporting Use of Lift Teams

Case Study	Description of Lift Teams	Outcomes
Woodland Healthcare; Charney (*J. Healthcare Safety*, Vol. 4, No. 3, 2000)	Crossed trained transport team	Restricted days reduced from 160 pre-lift team to 2 days post-lift team
"10 Hospital Study"; Charney (*AAOHN*, Vol. 4, No. 4, 1993)	23.9 combined years of data from 10 acute care facilities	90% decrease on lost days, 72% reduction in workers' compensation costs, and 69% reduction in injury rates
"18 Hospital Study"; Charney (*J. Healthcare Safety*, Vol. 1, No. 2, 2003)	18 acute care facilities	All 18 hospitals shared statistically significant reductions in all rates
Kaiser Permanente; California (Anecdotal: Memoranda from Safety Officer)	Kaiser California requires lift teams in all facilities	46% reduction in Kaiser hospitals using lift teams as an aggregate
Harborview Medical Ctr.; Seattle, Washington (Anecdotal: Information from Director of Program)	450-bed receiving acute care facility with lift teams 24/7	Lost days reduced from 1474 to 470 first year of implementation
Tri-City Health Systems, San Diego, California; Charney (Part of 10 Hospital Study cited above)	450-bed acute care facility with lift teams	Reduced workers' compensation costs from $247,000 to $14,000 and lost days from 788 to 0
Sutter Health Systems California; Donaldson (*J. Healthcare Safety*, Vol. 4, No. 2, 2000)	6 years of data	Reduction of frequency from 12.9 to 1.3 and indemnity reduction from 9.7 to 0.8
Sioux Valley Medical; Hefti, K. (*AAOHN*, Vol. 51, No. 6, June 2003)	600-bed acute care hospital	52% reduction lost days—1st year; 95% reduction lost days—2nd year

TABLE 8.1 *(Continued)*

Case Study	Description of Lift Teams	Outcomes
"10 Hospital Study"; Alaska Native Med. Ctr.; Charney (*J. Healthcare Safety*, Vol. 1, No. 2, 2003)	220-bed acute care	5-year data reduced lost time injury from 61/100 FTEs to 20/100 FTEs
Tampa General Hospital (Anecdotal information from workers' compensation Coordinator)	900-bed acute care/2 teams 7 days per week	2004—only one patient handling, lost time injury
Caska, B. (*AOHP Journal*, Spring 2000)	3 nursing homes	0 injuries on shifts using lift teams
University of WA Med. Ctr.; Davis, A. (*J. Healthcare Safety*, Vol. 4, No. 5, 2001)	350-bed acute care	85% reduction in lost days 1st year
University of Chicago Hospital (Anecdotal)	576-bed acute care—2 teams 7 days per week	40% reduction of injuries 1st year
Mayo Clinic; Meteineun, E. (*J. Healthcare Safety*, Vol. 3, No. 3, 9/1999)	1500-bed acute care	0 injuries on day shift covered by lift team. Restricted days reduced by 361%. Cost of back injuries reduced by $310,000
Mt. Diablo Healthcare; Muir, John, California (AMN Healthcare/Online Journal, 7/2004)	576-bed acute care	Reduction of claims for back injury; $475,000 since 2002

SUMMARY

The lift team model has been used successfully for the last decade in acute care hospitals. Data show reductions in injuries, as well as positive cost-benefits. The risk reduction model of putting "risk where it can be controlled" and that "lifting and transferring patients is a skill rather than a random task" has shown validity in the practice of busy acute care hospitals. Given all the variables within the paradigm of patient movement, the transferring of patients needs to be considered as a profession with a specialized skill set that cannot be applied successfully by busy nursing personnel. Second, the physical design and layout of acute care facilities create hazardous conditions within, for safe lifting and transferring; they include rooms too small, bathrooms not large enough to accommodate mechanical equipment, doors too small for bariatric patients, sharp angles, inclines, rugs, etc., all of which suggest a team approach to minimize the danger of exposing this population of nursing caregivers. Since it has been found in the American Nurses Association survey of 2001 that 88% of nurses think about leaving the profession due to the "physical demands" of the work, it is the responsibility of the health systems that employ them to reduce these physical work stresses. This author believes that any hospital greater than 105 beds would profit from this model.

ACKNOWLEDGMENT

Lift team pictures are courtesy of Oregon Health Science University Medical Center.

REFERENCES

American Nurses Association (ANA) (2001). NursingWorld Health and Safety Survey. Retrieved January 26, 2005, from http://nursingworld.org/surveys/index.htm#hssurvey

Caska, B. E., Patnode, R. E., & Clickner, D. (2000). Implementing and using a nurse staffed lift team: Preliminary findings. *AAOHN Journal, 20*(2), 42–45, 48.

Caska, B. A., Patnode, R. E., & Clickner, D. (1998). Feasibility of a nurse staffed lift team. *AAOHN Journal, 46*(6), 283–288.

Charney, W. (1992). The lifting team: second year data reported (News). *AAOHN Journal, 40*(10), 503.

Charney, W. (1997). The lift team method for reducing back injuries. A 10 hospital study. *AAOHN Journal, 45*(6), 300–304.

Charney, W. (2000). Reducing back injury in nursing cross training a transport team to be the lift team. *Journal of Healthcare Safety, 4*(3), 1–6.

Charney, W. (2003a). How to accomplish a responsible cost-benefit back injury analysis in the health care industry. In W. Charney, & A. Hudson (Eds.), *Back injury among healthcare workers* (pp. 41–47). Boca Raton, FL: CRC Press (Lewis Publishers).

Charney, W. (2003b). Preventing back injuries to healthcare workers using lift teams: data for 18 hospitals. *Journal of Healthcare Safety, 1*(2), 21–29.

Charney, W., Zimmerman, K., & Walara, E. (1991). The lifting team: a design method to reduce lost time back injury in nursing. *AAOHN Journal, 39*(5), 231–234.

Cohen-Mansfield, J., Culpepper, W. J., & Carter, P. (1996). Nursing staff back injuries: prevalence and cost in long term care facilities. *AAOHN Journal*, *44*(1), 9–17.

Davis, A. (1999). Birth of a lift team. *Journal of Healthcare Safety*, *5*(1), 15–18.

Donaldson, A. (2000). Lift team intervention: a six year picture. *Journal of Healthcare Safety*, *4*(2), 65–68.

Garg, A., Owen, B., & Carlson, B. (1992). Ergonomic evaluation of nursing assistants' jobs in a nursing home. *Ergonomics*, *35*(9), 979–995.

Haiduven, D. (2003). Lifting teams in health care facilities: a literature review. *AAOHN Journal*, *51*(5), 210–218.

Hefti, K. S., Farnham, R. J., Docken, L., Bentaas, R., Bossman, S., & Schaefer, J. (2003). Back injury prevention: a lift team success story. *AAOHN Journal*, *51*(6), 246–251.

McAbee, R., & Wilkinson, W. (1988). Back injuries and registered nurses. *AAOHN Journal*, *36*, 106–112.

Meittunen, E. J., Matzke, K., McCormack, H., & Sobczak, S. C. (1999). The effect of focusing ergonomic risk factors on a patient transfer team to reduce incidents among nurses associated with patient care. *Journal of Healthcare Safety, Compliance and Infection Control*, *2*(7), 306–312.

Nelson, A., & Fragala, G. (2003). Equipment for safe patient handling and movement. In W. Charney, & A. Hudson (Eds.), *Back injury among healthcare workers* (pp. 121–135). Boca Raton, FL: CRC Press (Lewis Publishers).

Owen, B. D., & Garg, A. (1992). Four methods for identification of most back stressing tasks. *International Journal of Economics*, *9*, 213–220.

Richards, B. (2005, in review). Internal Document. Ohio State University Medical Center.

Stobbe, T. J., & Plummer, R. W. (1988). Incidence of low back injuries among nursing personnel as a function of patient lifting frequency. *Journal of Safety Research*, *19*(1), 21–28.

Worthington, K. (2001). Stress and overwork top nurses concerns. *American Journal of Nursing*, *101*(12), 96.

CHAPTER NINE

Unit-Based Peer Safety Leaders to Promote Safe Patient Handling

Mary Matz

Historically, education and training approaches to decrease injuries from patient handling tasks have been largely ineffective. Three decades of education in body mechanics and training in lifting techniques have not turned the course for nursing injuries (Anderson, 1980; Brown, 1972; Buckle, 1981, 1987; Daws, 1981; Daltroy, Iversen, Larson, et al, 1997; Dehlin, Hedenrud, & Horal, 1976; Hayne, 1984; Harber et al., 1994; Lagerstrom & Hagberg, 1997; Larese & Fiorito, 1994; Owen & Garg, 1991; Shaw, 1981; Snook et al., 1978; St. Vincent, Tellier, & Lortie, 1989; Stubbs, Buckle, Hudson, & Rivers, 1983; Venning, 1988; Wood, 1987). As other vulnerable industries such as construction and farming have gradually decreased their frequency of injuries over time, nursing and personal care industries have maintained or increased (Figure 9.1). With the many years of body mechanics and proper lifting techniques training, in 2001, workers in nursing homes were twice as likely to be injured on the job than industry workers (13.9 injuries/100 full-time workers and 6.1 injuries/100 full-time injuries, respectively) (Bureau of

"The views expressed in this article are those of the author and do not necessarily represent the view of the Department of Veterans Affairs. No claim made to U.S. government material. Contact Author: Mary.Matz@med.va.gov."

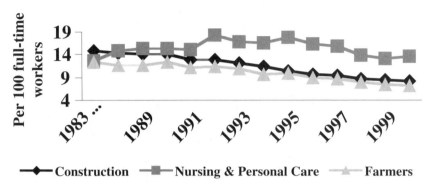

Source: US Department of Labor, Occupational Safety & Health Administration (2001).

FIGURE 9.1   Comparison of OSHA injury rates in nursing and industry.

Labor Statistics, 2002). Although proponents of these ineffective educational and training methods continue their promotion, there is a new and effective approach to decreasing nursing injuries in caregivers. This approach includes an ergonomic analysis of the work environment, the introduction of patient handling equipment, and critical support structures including a peer leader program. The value of this critical support structure lies in the roles of peer leaders as informal unit leaders, champions of safety, and facilitators of knowledge transfer. Knowledge transfer is essential for safe patient handling success and ranges from formal group education and training to informal one-on-one exchanges and brainstorming sessions. In facilitating such knowledge transfer, peer leaders "lead" by example, promote learning as a two-way street, and empower staff by placing value on the knowledge they possess.

WHAT IS A PEER SAFETY LEADER?

To be successful, the implementation of any new program necessitates a knowledgeable person with enthusiasm and leadership capabilities to direct and maintain the charge. Current management philosophy supports this use of peer safety leaders to effect change as well as increase staff involvement in management issues (Hammer & Champy, 1993). Patient care unit-based peer safety leaders provide these functions as well as others. They implement and maintain patient care ergonomic program elements, facilitate knowledge transfer on program elements and equipment, act as unit experts and resources on patient care ergonomics and equipment, champion the patient care ergonomic cause, and monitor and evaluate the program. They participate in or lead the unit ergonomic hazard evaluation to determine what patient handling equipment is warranted for their unit. Furthermore, they perform continual environmental hazard monitoring for ergonomic and other safety hazards. And, if that is not enough, they also train staff, implement equipment introduction, consult in new construction design, analyze facility injury data, and respond not only to ergonomic but to all safety concerns. A natural outcome of these unit peer leaders activities, a "Culture of Safety" is fostered to support clinicians in providing safe patient care and safe working environments.

KEY PROCESSES OF PEER SAFETY LEADERS

The two key processes integral to the performance of peer safety leaders are knowledge transfer and leadership. Each will be briefly described.

Knowledge Transfer

Knowledge transfer is essential for safe patient handling success and ranges from formal group education and training to informal one-on-one exchanges and brainstorming sessions. Any time knowledge is shared, knowledge transfer occurs. It promotes learning as a two-way street and empowers staff by placing value on the knowledge they possess. It is a way to share best practices and learn from mistakes.

Much knowledge generated in work settings is not shared and therefore is not usable. And, specific to healthcare, patient care ergonomic programs are not successful if designed without careful input and planning from direct care providers (Fragala & Bailey, 2003; Nelson et al., in review; US Department of Labor, OSHA, 2003; Yassi et al., 2001). Although ergonomic hazard evaluations may facilitate program success by identifying and controlling for risks in patient care environments, staff input is critical to supply specific information about their workplace. As well, frontline care providers know the true nature of risk embedded in their workplace (Fragala & Bailey, 2003; Nelson et al., in review) and this knowledge needs to be tapped. Programs designed in isolation often lead to costly mistakes and frustration when nurses do not use equipment and fail to embrace program elements. Staff input is necessary for making good equipment purchase decisions because of their knowledge of their patient population (Collins, Wolf, Bell, & Evanoff, 2004; Fragala & Bailey, 2003; Nelson, 2001; Nelson et al., in review).

For these reasons, effective methods of knowledge transfer, such as unit peer leaders, are essential to program success. In their many roles, peer leaders are conduits of information by sharing knowledge with and receiving information from co-workers, management, and other peer safety leaders.

Leadership

All people are potential leaders. Leaders do not have to hold a formal position of leadership or must they be perceived as a leader by others (House, 1997). Astin and Astin (1996) define a leader as ". . . one who is able to effect positive change for the betterment of others, the community, and society." The research of Bowers and Seashore (1996) established that leader behaviors can be shared by members of work units. They found use of peer leadership actually showed higher correlations with agency performance than formal manager leadership. Bowers and Seashore (1996) found peer leadership to be associated with a high level of organizational performance.

While more common in other industries, informal leadership positions can be found in healthcare. Although not formally labeled as such, hospital facility lead maintenance staff, lead engineering mechanics, charge nurses, etc. are utilized as peer safety leaders to increase staff involvement in management and/or assist supervisors in their roles. This innovative use of staff as leaders effectively demonstrates the OSHA Ergonomic Guidelines for Nursing Homes (2003) suggestion that employee involvement enhances worker motivation and job satisfaction, and leads to greater acceptance when changes are made in the workplace (US Department of Labor, OSHA, 2003). Healthcare-focused researchers have noted that organizational performance may be affected by increased staff involvement and support of program goals. One reason is that peer safety leaders forge a direct connection between staff and program goals by fostering knowledge transfer (Nelson, 2001; Pillemer, Meador, Hoffman, & Schumacher, 2001). In their VHA sponsored research project, *VISN-Wide Deployment of a Back Injury Prevention Program for Nurses: Safe Patient Handling and Movement*, Nelson et al. (in review) noted that the VHA peer safety leaders were prime examples of how to garner nursing support and sustain program benefits over time (Nelson, 2001; Nelson et al., in review).

OPERATIONALIZING PEER SAFETY LEADERS

VHA investigators realized the need for knowledge transfer conduits and facilitators. They included peer safety leaders, which they called BIRNs (Back Injury Resource Nurses), to empower nurses to promote safety in their workplace. The VHA unit peer safety leader model initially included one peer safety leader, or BIRN, per high-risk unit involved in the study. The VHA BIRNs were considered informal leaders who were respected by co-workers. BIRNs drove the program from inception and continually thereafter. They facilitated implementation of the ergonomics system approach, no-lift policy, assessment and algorithms for safe patient handling, After Action Review (AAR) process, and competency assessments related to safe use of equipment. The BIRNs were linked electronically and promoted knowledge transfer within and across sites by participating in weekly facility meetings and region-wide semi-monthly conference calls. They still offer customized knowledge transfer that is tailored to address unique characteristics and conditions of their unit. BIRNs provide safe patient handling expertise, meet with co-workers individually or in groups, provide ongoing hazard identification, and assure staff competency in equipment use and use of algorithms. They demonstrate use of equipment and problem-solve issues associated with implementation. As champions of safety and staff empowerment, they facilitate creation of an effective culture of safety on their units.

The VHA safe patient handling and movement program that included BIRN unit peer safety leaders successfully showed significant decreases in injury rates and modified duty days. Job satisfaction indices, perception of professional status and task requirements, increased significantly after the intervention was instituted. Focus group participants noted that the constant support of BIRN nurses, new equipment, and staff training boosted staff morale. Overall, the role of the BIRN was deemed quite effective and most managers stressed the desire for the BIRNs to maintain visibility and availability and interact with nursing staff during patient handling and movement tasks after the study was terminated. At the end of the VHA study, the level of perceived support for BIRNs was almost 100% from co-workers, management, and patients. Managers also felt there was a positive impact on nursing satisfaction and therefore retention, as well as on recruitment.

BJC Healthcare instituted the use of a somewhat similar successful peer safety leader model, Ergo Rangers. They are facility-wide rather than unit-based, but, in patient care settings, the role of the ergo ranger mirrors that of BIRNs. These individuals provide expertise and support to patient care staff in proper patient handling techniques and use of equipment. They train staff and implement the use of new equipment. Different from the BIRNs, they provide support to other hospital employees on global ergonomic issues, perform injury data analysis to identify ergonomic problem areas, and act as consultants for new construction design. Recently, BJC Healthcare instituted a BIRN/Ergo Ranger combo. An Ergo Ranger turned RN became the nurse advocate for ergonomics on her unit but Ergo Rangers still assist her in training and equipment issues. A physical therapist with ergonomics training is also assigned to the same floor. Anecdotally, the result of this model has been quite positive, with evidence of increased usage of lifting equipment (Matz & Wolf, 2004).

In the Netherlands, a highly successful peer safety leader program is given responsibility for initiating and ensuring that ergonomic changes take place that provide safer patient care environments. At this writing there are nearly 10,000 ErgoCoaches in the Netherlands and the program is rapidly expanding (Knibbe, 2005). Knibbe & Knibbe (2005) found that facilities with ErgoCoaches have significantly lower sick leave due to musculoskeletal disorders and assert that the synergy between the work of thousands of ErgoCoaches, the ErgoCoach National Support Group, and governmental working condition covenants was key to this success (Knibbe & Knibbe, n.d.). One or two of these ErgoCoaches are found on every participating ward. As a unit peer leader, an ErgoCoach takes responsibility not only as the problem-owner but also as the solution-owner. The rationale is that these unit-based leaders know first hand the issues on the unit and the corresponding needs, and, with comprehensive training, are empowered to foster safer work environments. As with BIRNs and Ergo Rangers, ErgoCoaches are the unit ergonomic experts and provide training and updates on equipment and ergonomic issues of interest. They are informal leaders that can interact easily with co-workers and have good communications skills, a fundamental to success according to Knibbe and Knibbe (n.d.). Appreciating the importance for such communication conduits or knowledge transfer mechanisms, the Netherlands government established an ErgoCoach National Support Group to ensure that ErgoCoaches are provided with the most current ergonomic information and technology for healthcare environments. Networking and knowledge transfer between ErgoCoaches is of high priority for this organization, so ErgoCoach members are provided a help desk, website, newsletter, and an annual conference where thousands of ErgoCoaches convene. ErgoCoaches are actively supported in their efforts not only nationally but also at the facility level.

TOOLS AND STRATEGIES FOR IMPLEMENTATION

Selection Criteria

Candidates must be considered "informal" leaders on their unit. They must be respected by their co-workers for their nursing skills and based on their personal merit. Good time management skills are important. Nurse managers can select peer leaders or draw from a pool of volunteers.

Selection should not be limited to Registered Nurses (RNs). Any interested staff member should have the potential to be selected; however, it has been found that RNs with other leadership responsibilities have more flexibility in their schedules, allowing for more consistency in availability and fulfillment of their roles. Ergonomic experience is not required, but candidates must be motivated, enthusiastic, and assertive (Matz & Wolf, 2004).

Coverage/Time Requirements

Initially, in the VHA program, one peer leader was selected for each high-risk unit. Over time, though, many of these units brought in additional peer leaders in an attempt to cover all shifts and as many staff as possible. Units that opted to assign peer leaders on each shift noted benefits of increased visibility and timeliness of training. These "unit-based" peer leaders performed their duties as a collateral assignment, maintaining patient care responsibilities as well. In contrast, other facilities have found that one full-time peer leader for an entire facility was effective (Matz & Wolf, 2004).

Training

The unit peer leader role is not static. It requires continued exposure to new strategies to maintain safe work environments. The work environment of nurses is unique, combining high levels of ergonomic risk and environmental hazards; consequently, ongoing training is a must. For instance, equipment training should occur whenever new equipment is introduced. In order to fulfill their role, peer leaders must be knowledgeable of adult education philosophies and be able to coach and motivate co-workers as well as assess workplace hazards and maintain safe work environments. Training programs vary in content and time, but generally include evidence-based patient care ergonomics and the rationale for and use of program elements such as After Action Review and patient handling algorithms. And importantly, classes in how to train, coach, and motivate co-workers are included. In instances when existing peer safety leaders are unable to fulfill their roles, other facility unit peer leaders mentor new ones until formal training can be accomplished. Mentoring programs for new peer safety leaders facilitate socialization to the role. Even with formal training, unit peer leaders are continually learning, from each other, from their peers, from equipment companies, etc. Beyond the initial and annual training provided to the BIRNS in the VHA program, much of the ongoing training was primarily "on-the-job." (Matz & Wolf, 2004).

Administrative Support

As with any program and program element, administrative support is crucial for success. Management must allow unit peer leaders to perform their role as required. This means support of safe patient handling and movement education and training for peer leaders as well as assistance with peer leader's training role. And importantly, management must allocate adequate time to carry out their responsibilities. Mangers who actively utilize unit peer leaders as resources for patient handling themselves provide a role model for their staff. Management will benefit from support of a peer leader role. As noted previously, at the end of the VHA study, managers felt there was a positive impact on nursing satisfaction, thus retention and recruitment.

Knowledge Transfer

With patient care ergonomic knowledge in hand, it is important for peer safety leaders to be able to share their knowledge and experience. They train, act as resources for, and coach co-workers. Unit-based peer safety leaders share their knowledge on program elements and equipment with co-workers through in-services and during competency training. They promote knowledge transfer among staff through the use of AAR. On the job, they communicate patient care ergonomic information to co-workers and new staff.

Facility-based peer safety leaders facilitate knowledge transfer within their group during weekly team meetings and by participating in departmental training using observation and critique methods. They conduct "train-the-trainer" sessions to facilitate knowledge transfer to others in their facilities. Knowledge-based information is relayed during staff meetings, and skill-based/hands-on learning is completed individually. On-the-job training is commonly used for new and existing employees, and while these peer leaders perform their unit ergonomic and safety inspections, they provide this expertise to others. To lighten competency evaluations, they hold "competency days" to establish staff competency in patient care ergonomics and equipment use (Matz & Wolf, 2004). Minimally, monthly face-to-face or conference call meetings should be held to share new information, assist with problem solving, and provide support.

Generally, the most successful methods of knowledge transfer of patient care ergonomic information in patient care environments include the following methods. (1) *Demonstration* is a hands-on training method that shows how equipment or a program element actually works and procedures for use. (2) *Competency-based training* is based on the demonstration method but includes assessments to assure accuracy in performing activities. (3) *Brainstorming* facilitates the free flow of ideas stimulating creative thinking and development of new ideas, and ease in sharing knowledge and ideas. (4) *Peer-to-peer knowledge transfer* allows co-workers to learn from one another and facilitates knowledge of specific unit idiosyncrasies to be incorporated in the learning process. It empowers those involved as does mentorship. (5) *Mentorship* is informal guidance from one who is knowledgeable to one who desires to learn more. It has the benefit of focusing on topics/activities that are relevant and of most importance to the learner.

STRATEGIES FOR SUCCESS

- *Implementation in high-risk units.* This intervention is probably most applicable for high-risk units because peer safety leaders are resource intensive, in that they require continued education and exposure to new strategies to maintain safe work environments, and success is dependent on the support of management and administration at all levels.
- *Management support prior to institution of peer leader program.* The degree of unit peer leader success is limited by the degree of management support. Peer safety leaders must have management backing in order for his/her peers to recognize the role as essential and worthwhile.
- *Comprehensive training program.* Training is critical to support program elements and equipment use. Support from nurse educators is essential assisting peer leaders in training staff and other such duties. Providing a train-the-trainer method of training may lighten training responsibilities. Modified duty staff may also be helpful.
- *Time to perform the role of unit peer safety leader.* Sufficient time must be allowed for the peer leaders to carry out expected activities.
- *Incentives for peer leaders.* Offer incentives to peer leaders who demonstrate excellent performance.
- *Commitment to education and training.* Commit to ongoing unit safety peer leader education through conference attendance, equipment manufacturer training, and other applicable training/education.

CASE SCENARIO

A BIRN on a VHA Spinal Cord Injury Unit noted that the friction-reducing devices (FRDs) purchased for her unit were not being used by the staff. They were purchased to reduce loads during lateral transfers and resulting musculoskeletal injuries. From her BIRN training, she knew the dangers inherent in performing lateral transfers manually with no assistive device, so she held an AAR (see Chapter 7) on the subject with her co-workers. During the AAR, it was determined that staff were not using the new FRDs because they were too narrow for their generally large male patients. The BIRN contacted the manufacturer and discussed the problem. The manufacturer agreed to produce wider FRDs, and after their introduction, staff used them regularly. She shared this information during a weekly facility BIRN meeting and during a regional BIRN teleconference, so other BIRNs were able to determine if this situation was a problem for their units. The BIRNs expertise in patient care ergonomics and the understanding of the merit of knowledge transfer reduced risk for musculoskeletal injury both on her unit and in other patient care units within the region.

REFERENCES

Anderson, J. (1980). Back pain and occupation. In M. I. V. Jayson (Ed.), *The lumbar spine and back pain* (2nd ed., pp. 57–82). London: Pitman Medical Ltd.

Astin, H. S., & Astin, A. W. (1996). *A social change model of leadership development guidebook, version 3*. Los Angeles, CA: Higher Education Research Institute, University of California, Los Angeles.

Bowers, D. G., & Seashore, S. E. (1966). Predicting organizational effectiveness with a four-factor theory of leadership. *Administrative Science Quarterly, 11*, 238–263.

Brown, J. (1972). Minimal lifting and related fields. An annotated bibliography. Labor Safety Council of Ontario.

Buckle, P. (1981). A multidisciplinary investigation of factors associated with low back pain. PhD Thesis, Cranfield Institute of Technology.

Buckle, P. (1987). Epidemiological aspects of back within the nursing profession. *International Journal of Nursing Studies, 24*(4), 319–324.

Bureau of Labor Statistics (2002). Survey of occupational inquiries and illnesses, 2001. US Department of Labor. USDL December 19, 2002.

Collins, J. W., Wolf, L., Bell, J., & Evanoff, B. (2004). An evaluation of a "best practices" musculoskeletal injury prevention program in nursing homes. *Injury Prevention, 10*(4), 206–11.

Daltroy, L. H., Iversen, M. D., Larson, M. G., Lew, R., Wright, E., Ryan, J., Zwerling, C., Fossel, A. H., & Liang, M. H. (1997). A controlled trial of an educational program to prevent low back injuries. *The New England Journal of Medicine, 337*(5), 322–328.

Daws, J. (1981). Lifting and moving patients, 3, a revision training programme. *Nursing Times, 77*(48), 2067–2069.

Dehlin, O., Hedenrud, B., & Horal, J. (1976). Back symptoms in nursing assistants in a geriatric hospital. *Scandinavian Journal of Rehabilitation Medicine, 8*(2), 47–53.

Fragala, G., & Bailey, L. P. (2003). Addressing occupational strains and sprains: musculoskeletal injuries in hospitals. *AAOHN Journal, 51*(6), 252–259.

Harber, P., Pena, L., Hsu, P., Billet, E., Greer, D., & Kim, K. (1994). Personal history, training and worksite as predictors of back pain in nurses. *American Journal of Industrial Medicine, 25*, 519–526.

Hammer, M., & Champy, J. (1993). *Reengineering the corporation: A manifesto for business revolution*. New York: Harper Business.

Hayne, C. (1984). Ergonomics and back pain. *Physiotherapy, 70*(1), 9–13.

Hignett, S., Crumpton, E., Ruszala, S., Alexander, P., Fray, M., & Fletcher, B. (2003). *Evidence-based patient handling: Tasks, equipment and interventions*. New York: Routledge.

House, R. J. (1997). The social scientific study of leadership: Quo Vadis? *Journal of Management, 23*(3), 409.

Knibbe, H. (2005). *Ergonomic Approach in the Netherlands: Experience*. Presentation at the 5th Annual Safe Patient Handling and Movement Conference, St. Pete Beach, FL.

Knibbe, H., & Knibbe, N. (n.d.). Solving back pain in the health care industry: The Dutch approach. Retrieved July 27, 2005 from http://www.arbo.nl/news/conference_docs/proceedings/GBIII/sessie5/Knibbe.doc

Lagerstrom, M., & Hagberg, M. (1997). Evaluation of a 3 year education and training program for nursing personnel at a Swedish hospital. *AAOHN Journal, 45*(2), 83–92.

Larese, F., & Fiorito, A. (1994). Musculoskeletal disorders in hospital nurses: a comparison between two hospitals. *Ergonomics, 37*(7), 1205–1211.

Matz, M., & Wolf, L. (2004). *Peer leaders as a new education strategy*. Presentation at the 4th Annual Safe Patient Handling and Movement Conference, Orlando, FL.

Nelson, A. (Ed.). (2001). Patient care ergonomics resource guide: Safe patient handling and movement. Retrieved July 20, 2004 from http://www.patientsafetycenter.com/Safe%20Pt%20Handling%20Div.htm

Nelson, A., Matz, M., Chen, F., Siddharthan, K., Lloyd, J., & Fragala, G. (in review). Development and Evaluation of a Multifaceted Ergonomics Program To Prevent Injuries Associated with Patient Handling Tasks. *International Journal of Nursing Studies*.

Owen, B., & Garg, A. (1991). Reducing the risk for back pain in nursing personnel. *AAOHN Journal, 39*, 24–33.

Pillemer, K., Meador, R., Hoffman, R., & Schumacher, M. (2001). Retrieved July 20, 2004 from http://www.frontlinepub.com/pdf/MentorSample.pdf

Shaw, R. (1981). Creating back care awareness. *Dimensions in Health Service, 58*(3), 32–33.

Snook, S., Campanelli, R., & Hart, J. (1978). A study of three preventive approaches to low back injury. *Journal of Occupational Medicine, 20*(7), 478–481.

St. Vincent, M., Tellier, C., & Lortie, M. (1989). Training in handling: an evaluative study. *Ergonomics, 32*(2), 191–210.

Stubbs, D., Buckle, P, Hudson, M., & Rivers, P. (1983). Back pain in the nursing profession. II. The effectiveness of training. *Ergonomics, 26*(8), 767–779.

US Department of Labor, Occupational Safety and Health Administration. (2003). Ergonomic Guidelines for Nursing Homes. Retrieved July 20, 2004 from http://www.osha.gov/ergonomics/guidelines/nursinghome/final_nh_guidelines.html. Accessibility verified.

Venning, P. (1988). Back injury prevention among nursing personnel. *AAOHN Journal, 36*(8), 327–333.

Wood, D. (1987). Design and evaluation of a back injury prevention program within a geriatric hospital. *Spine, 12*(2), 77–82.

Yassi, A., Cooper, J. E., Tate, R. B., Gerlach, S., Muir, M., Trottier, J., & Massey, K. (2001). A randomized controlled trial to prevent patient lift and transfer injuries of health care workers. *Spine, 26*(16), 1739–1746.

CHAPTER TEN

Safe Lifting Policies

James W. Collins

A safe-lifting policy (also referred to as "no-lift," "zero-lift," "minimal-lift," "no-manual-lift," or a "safe patient lifting policy") is one part of a comprehensive approach to preventing musculoskeletal injuries to healthcare workers. The purpose of a written safe-lifting policy is to provide a clear understanding of the elements of a safe patient handling and movement program, to define the roles and responsibilities for all affected staff (healthcare administrators, supervisors, frontline caregivers, therapy staff, maintenance personnel, and housekeeping staff) and to provide a reference for review when questions arise.

The policy provides guidance for assessing the transferring needs of patients and for the training requirements to ensure the appropriate use of lifting equipment and repositioning aids. In addition, guidance is provided for staff responsibilities, equipment storage and maintenance, and the resources required to purchase and maintain the lifting equipment, and other assistive devices. The basic premise of a safe-lifting policy is to avoid the manual handling of patients wherever possible; manual handling is defined as "the transporting or supporting of a patient by hand or bodily force, including pushing, pulling, carrying, holding, and supporting of the patient or a body part" (Royal College of Nursing Code of Practice for Patient Handling 2000).

"The findings and conclusions in this chapter are those of the author(s) and do not necessarily represent the views of the National Institute for Occupational Safety and Health."

Because safe-lifting policies are not mandated in the United States, the State of Texas passed the first state law requiring hospitals and nursing homes to implement a safe patient handling and movement program as of January 1, 2006. Misconceptions have impeded the widespread implementation of safe-lifting policies and safe patient handling and movement programs in hospitals and nursing homes. Common misconceptions about safe-lifting policies include: (a) caregivers should never attempt to lift or move a patient; (b) nurses should not use lift equipment; and (c) the policy only applies to high-risk tasks associated with patient lifts, and ignores other high-risk tasks such as repositioning patients in beds and chairs (Nelson & Baptiste, 2004). A written safe-lifting policy can overcome many of the barriers and misconceptions by clearly describing the responsibilities of each member of the healthcare team, equipment and training requirements, and procedures necessary to safely lift and move patients. Research in diverse healthcare settings (private, non-profit, and government-owned hospitals, and long-term care facilities) has demonstrated that safe-lifting policies can be highly effective for reducing the risk of injury to both caregivers and patients (Collins, Wolf, Bell, & Evanoff, 2004; Garg, 1999; Garg & Owen, 1992; Nelson & Fragala, 2004; Nelson, Fragala, & Menzel, 2003; Yassi et al., 2001).

HISTORY OF SAFE-LIFTING PROGRAMS

In comparison to the limited implementation of safe-lifting policies and safe patient handling and movement programs in the United States, hospitals, nursing homes, and community healthcare settings in the United Kingdom have been legally required to comply with a safe-lifting policy under the Manual Handling Operations Regulations since 1992. The United Kingdom policy requires that, "the manual lifting of patients should be eliminated in all but exceptional or life threatening situations" (Royal College of Nursing Code of Practice for Patient Handling, 2000) and "patients should be encouraged to assist in their own transfers and handling aids must be used whenever they can help to reduce risk if this is not contrary to a patient's needs. It is important to avoid any handling which involves manually lifting most or all of a patient's weight." It is acceptable to give a patient some support, or to perform horizontal moves with a sliding aid, if done according to agreed safe handling principles. The United Kingdom policy does not specify a weight limit. The main message of the policy is that staff should not attempt to lift any patients manually, whatever their weight, except in hospital units which deal with babies and small children.

Similar regulations have been adopted in Australia and Canada (Australian Nursing Federation, 1998; Workers' Compensation Board of British Columbia, 2004). The Australian Nursing Federation adopted the Royal College of Nursing's definition of a safe-lifting policy (Australian Nursing Federation No Lift Policy, 1998). The Australian and Canadian policies promote the use of mechanical lifting aids and other equipment to assist nursing staff with moving, transferring, and handling of patients to ensure that minimal force is exerted by caregivers when handling patients. Patients are encouraged to assist in their own transfers and handling aids must be used whenever they can help to reduce risk, as long as this is not contrary to a patient's needs.

CORE ELEMENTS OF A SAFE-LIFTING POLICY

A safe-lifting policy should address the following points, but may include additional provisions depending on the patient transferring needs of the healthcare facility:

- Purpose of the safe-lifting policy
- The program's goals for reducing worker musculoskeletal injuries and improving the quality of patient care
- Workplace injury and environmental assessment to determine equipment requirements and potential workplace modifications
- Methods for assessing the transferring needs of each patient (refer to the algorithms in Chapter 5) and determining the safest techniques for lifting and moving patients
- Resources available for lifting equipment, repositioning aids, and bathing equipment that will be required to establish a safe patient handling and movement program
- Roles and responsibilities of the administrator, nurse managers, maintenance and housekeeping staff, and frontline caregivers who perform patient lifting
- Training and education requirements for affected staff (caregivers, administrators, nurse managers, therapy staff, and maintenance and housekeeping staff)
- Infection control issues
- Equipment maintenance schedules and procedures
- Equipment storage and battery charging procedures
- Procedures and equipment for handling bariatric and other special needs patients
- Procedures for evacuating patients in an emergency

PURPOSE OF THE SAFE-LIFTING POLICY

The purpose of the safe-lifting policy is to prevent injuries associated with patient lifting and to provide clearly written guidelines for safe patient lifting that explains the roles and responsibilities of all staff affected by the policy. Adherence to the policy should ensure that the transferring needs of all patients have been assessed and all affected staff are aware of the policy requirements and all healthcare staff responsible for transferring patients have been trained on the correct procedures to transfer each patient.

SETTING GOALS AND OBJECTIVES

The initial review of the injury data can be used to establish baseline measures of the frequency and severity of injuries, the number of days away from work and restricted workdays, and determine injury-related costs associated with patient handling incidents. These baseline measures can be used to target injury prevention efforts, establish goals and objectives for reducing injuries to staff and patients, and provide a benchmark to measure the impact of the program.

WORKPLACE INJURY AND ENVIRONMENTAL ASSESSMENT

Prior to the development of a safe-lifting policy and a safe patient lifting program, a review of the injuries to staff and patients associated with patient handling and an assessment of the patient care environment should be conducted by a site visit team who understands the ergonomic processes specific to patient care environments. Site visit team members should include key staff from the unit, such as the nurse manager, supervisor, and nursing staff and persons with training in ergonomics such as Industrial Hygienists, Occupational Medicine Practitioners, or Ergonomists.

A review of the injury data and injury-related costs (workers' compensation, OSHA logs, and occupational health logs) can help identify high-risk units. A review and analysis of the injury data can identify who is being injured (patients and/or staff), how they are being injured, where these injuries are occurring, the circumstances under which the injuries occur, how serious the injuries are, how many injuries are occurring and over what time period, and provide insight as to how the injuries might be prevented. An environmental assessment should examine the layout of patient rooms, bathrooms, and bathing areas to identify factors that contribute to patient handling incidents such as furniture that might interfere with transfers; the adjustability of bed height; the size of the bathrooms and bathing areas; and thresholds that are not level with the floor that might create barriers for lifting equipment. This baseline information can be used to justify allocation of resources to establish a safe patient lifting program, identify the type of equipment that can be used to lift and move patients, and to establish goals for injury and cost reduction. Baseline information provides a benchmark against which to measure the effectiveness of the safe patient lifting program.

ASSESSING THE TRANSFERRING NEEDS OF EACH PATIENT

One of the most important elements of a safe-lifting policy is to provide direction on how to assess each patient's transferring needs and to prescribe lifting and transferring method(s) based on the patient's rehabilitation goals, ability to ambulate, bear weight, and follow verbal instructions. Chapter 5 provides a detailed discussion on how to use patient algorithms to assess a patient's transferring needs and how to prescribe the most appropriate methods to lift and move the patient.

RESOURCE ALLOCATION

There is fierce competition for resources in healthcare settings. Cost–benefit analyses have demonstrated that the initial investment in lifting equipment and employee training can be recovered in 2–3 years by the reduced workers' compensation costs attributed to these programs while concurrently improving the quality of patient care and caregiver safety (Collins et al., 2004; Garg, 1999; Nelson et al., 2003; Tiesman, Nelson, Charney, Siddharthan, & Fragala, 2003). The fact that safe patient lifting programs can recover the initial capital investment through reduced injury costs, improved worker safety and quality of patient care is persuasive evidence for influencing healthcare decision makers to allocate resources to establish and fund a safe patient handling and movement program.

ROLES AND RESPONSIBILITIES OF ALL STAFF

The roles and responsibilities of the administrator, physical and occupational therapists, charge nurses, nursing staff and other frontline caregivers, maintenance staff, and the housekeeping staff should be delineated in the safe-lifting policy.

EDUCATION AND TRAINING

A safe-lifting policy can increase compliance to safe patient lifting programs by specifying training requirements for all affected staff and by maintaining records of staff training. Numerous studies have shown that training caregivers to use proper body mechanics when lifting patients is not an effective prevention measure (Daltroy et al., 1997; Lagerstrom & Hagberg, 1997; Nelson et al., 2003); however, a safe patient lifting program that provides training to caregivers on how to assess the transferring needs of patients and how to use mechanical lifts and other equipment/aids is an effective prevention measure (Collins, Wolf, Bell, & Evanoff, 2004; Nelson & Fragala, 2004; Yassi et.al, 2001). When lifting equipment and repositioning aids are introduced in a healthcare facility, caregivers may be resistant to change and reluctant to adopt new methods of lifting and moving patients. Providing training and education to all staff affected by the program to inform them about the objectives of the program and their responsibilities and of their employer's commitment to the program can promote widespread support of the patient lifting program.

When equipment is initially purchased, the manufacturer generally provides training by a highly skilled individual with extensive knowledge of the equipment. However, because this individual may not be available for follow-up training, it is important that in-house staff become proficient in providing ongoing training for the healthcare facility. Training should be administered to all new hires annually and when new equipment or lifting practices are introduced.

It can be helpful if trainers are peer leaders from patient care areas who know the routine, patient needs, and techniques used in that area. Trainers can then lead by example, assess competence of newly trained staff, and monitor compliance in their work area. To enhance the effectiveness of the training program, staff designated as trainers should possess good interpersonal and communication skills and have the ability to design, deliver, and evaluate training and education programs.

The safe-lifting policy can also provide important details on how the training will be conducted, such as the maximum number of trainees per session and methods of training. Smaller classes facilitate more participation and provide trainees with essential hands-on practice. It is important for trainees to learn how to assess patients and to demonstrate competency in correctly using mechanical patient lifting equipment and other assistive devices. The competency process should be documented by the unit manager who is most familiar with the transferring needs of patients or by a certified trainer who shadows the employees on the unit.

INFECTION CONTROL CONSIDERATIONS

Infection control standards and procedures should be addressed in the safe-lifting policy. All patient lifting equipment, slings, and assistive devices should be cleaned and laundered to comply with infection control procedures and policies. Disposable slings should be used on patients who pose an infection control risk. If reusable slings are dedicated for use by specific patients or by certain units, marking the patients' name and/or their unit name on the sling and storing them at their bedside will also reduce the risk of losing slings during the laundering process. Patient lifting equipment should be cleaned on a regular basis and after each use with a patient who poses an infection control risk.

MAINTENANCE SCHEDULE AND PROCEDURES

Maintenance personnel should be trained how to inspect and perform routine repairs on lifting equipment, slings, and repositioning aids. The safe-lifting policy can specify the frequency and points of inspection, the process for making repairs and procedures for removing damaged equipment from service.

EQUIPMENT STORAGE AND BATTERY CHARGING PROCEDURES

One of the challenges of a safe patient lifting program is where to store lifting equipment and assistive devices so that equipment is readily accessible to staff. Storage may not be a problem for ceiling-mounted hoists that are stored overhead, but a careful assessment of the facility may be required to identify the best place to store portable equipment. Battery charging procedures should be specified in the lifting policy.

SUMMARY

In the absence of regulations that mandate safe-lifting policies or the use of mechanical equipment to lift and transfer patients at national or state levels (except Texas state legislation requiring safe patient handling and movement programs effective January 1, 2006), healthcare facilities must embrace proactive approaches to control ergonomic hazards in healthcare settings and prevent back injuries among the nation's healthcare workforce. Research has shown that safe-lifting policies are an essential part of safe patient handling and movement programs and can be highly effective for reducing the risk of injury to frontline caregivers while improving the quality of patient care. A safe-lifting policy and safe patient handling and movement program can reduce the physical stresses of nursing work, improve retention of healthcare staff by reducing the number of nurses leaving the profession due to back pain, and improve the quality of the lives of healthcare workers by reducing injury, sick leave, and fatigue.

CREATING A SAFE-LIFTING POLICY FOR A HEALTHCARE FACILITY

To help facilitate the development of a safe-lifting policy in a healthcare facility, a template is included in Appendix A located at the end of this chapter. A team approach is suggested to develop and implement a safe patient lifting policy. The team should have representatives from each department affected by the policy. The team should include, but not be limited to, facility managers, caregivers responsible for lifting and moving patients, staff from the physical/occupational therapy departments, maintenance and housekeeping management.

REFERENCES

Australian Nursing Federation (Victorian Branch) No Lift Policy, 1998. Retrieved July 26 (2004) from http://www.sa.anf.org.au/guest/benefits/ohs.asp

Collins, J. W., Wolf, L., Bell, J., & Evanoff, B. (2004). An evaluation of a "best practices" musculoskeletal injury prevention program in nursing homes. *Injury Prevention, 10,* 206–211.

Daltroy, L. H., Iverson, M. D., Larson, M. G., Lew, R., Wright, E., Ryan, J., Zwerling, C., Fossel, A. H., & Liang, M. H. (1997). A controlled trial of an educational program to prevent low back injuries. *New England Journal of Medicine, 337*(5), 322–328.

Garg, A. (1999). Long-term effectiveness of "zero-lift program" in seven nursing homes and one hospital. Contract No. U60/CCU512089-02. Accessed on October 25, 2004 at http://www.cdc.gov/nioshtic

Garg, A., & Owen, B. D. (1992). Reducing back stress to nursing personnel: an ergonomics intervention in a nursing home. *Ergonomics, 35*, 1353–1375.

Lagerstrom, M., & Hagberg, M. (1997). Evaluation of a 3-year education and training program. For nursing personnel at a Swedish hospital. *American Association of Occupational Health Nurses Journal, 45*(2), 83–92.

Nelson, A., & Baptiste, A. S. (2004). Evidence-based practices for safe patient handling and movement. *Online Journal of Issues in Nursing, 9*(3), Manuscript 3. Accessible online at: www.nursingworld.org/ojin/topic25/tpc_3/htm

Nelson, A., & Fragala, G. (2004). Equipment for safe patient handling and movement. In W. Charney, & A. Hudson (Eds.), *Back injury among Healthcare workers: Causes, solutions, and impacts* (pp. 121–135). Boca Raton, FL: Lewis Publishers.

Nelson, A., Fragala, G., & Menzel, N. (2003). Myths and facts about back injuries in nursing. *American Journal of Nursing, 103*(2), 32–40.

Nelson, A., Matz, M., Chen, F., Siddharthan, K., Lloyd, J., & Fragala, G. (2003). Research report: A multifaceted ergonomics program to prevent injuries associated with patient handling tasks in the Veteran's Hospital Association.

Royal College of Nursing (2000) *Code of Practice for Patient Handling.* Royal College of Nursing, England.

Tiesman, H., Nelson, A., Charney, W., Siddharthan, K., & Fragala, G. (2003). Effectiveness of a ceiling-mounted patient lift system in reducing occupational injuries in long-term care. *Journal of Healthcare Safety, 1*(1), 34–40.

Worksafe (Workers' Compensation Board of BC) (2004). *Handle with care: Patient handling and the application of ergonomics (MSI) requirements.* Retrieved March 12, 2004 from http://www.worksafebc.com

Yassi, A., Cooper, J. E., Tate, R. B., Gerlach, S., Muir, M., Trottier, J., & Massey, K. (2001). A randomized controlled trial to prevent patient lift and transfer injuries of healthcare workers. *Spine, 26*(16), 1739–1746.

Special Challenges in Patient Handling

CHAPTER ELEVEN

Preventing Injuries When Taking Care of Special Needs Patients

Hans-Peter de Ruiter and MaryAnn Burke de Ruiter

Previous chapters described concepts of the etiology and epidemiology of occupational injuries associated with patient handling, as well as ergonomic principles for assessing risk. Several evidence-based strategies to prevent patient handling injuries were delineated. These strategies have been deemed to be effective with most patients. However, special patient care populations exist, which offer unique challenges for safe patient handling and movement. This chapter focuses on seven special patient populations, including bariatrics, those with combative behaviors, cognitive impairments, severe pain, extensive wounds, or neurological conditions, as well as pediatric patients. The content is intended to build on the content discussed in the other chapters rather than to replace that content.

THE BARIATRIC PATIENT

Introduction

Risks associated with patient handling and movement are magnified when the patient is morbidly obese (Barr & Cunneen, 2001). Bariatrics refers to the care of patients who are morbidly obese (Nelson, Baptiste, de Ruiter, Thomason, & Belwood, in press), that is, persons who have a body mass index (BMI) greater than 30 (Centers for Disease Control, 2002).

Safely performing patient handling tasks for a morbidly obese patient provides significant challenges (Allison & Saunders, 2002; Kuczmarski & Flegal, 2000; Meittunen, Matzke, & Sobczak, 1999; Meittunen, McCormack, & Sobczak, 2000; Must et al., 1999; Youngkin & Kissinger, 1999). Beyond the obvious issues associated with body weight, the bariatric patient often has atypical body mass, uneven weight distribution, and multiple co-morbidities, which affect the way a patient handling task is performed. Specifically, the following patient factors contribute to the challenges in providing safe patient care (Baptiste, Meittunen & Bertschinger, 2004; Nelson et al., in press):

- Limitations in mobility (e.g., limited weight-bearing capacity)
- Poor respiratory status (e.g., decreased lung capacity)
- Mental health issues (e.g., depression)
- Impaired skin condition (e.g., cellulitis)
- Discomfort or pain (e.g., musculoskeletal pain)
- Barriers to discharge planning (e.g., inadequate access to housing or social support)

Assessment

The accurate assessment of bariatric patients is the key to preventing injuries in healthcare providers (Dionne, 2005). Solely looking at a patient's weight can easily lead to an inaccurate risk assessment resulting in an inadequate care plan. The key factors that should be assessed are:

- *Body mass index (BMI):* The BMI can be calculated by dividing the patient's weight (in kg) by the patient's height squared (in m^2). Many BMI calculators can be found online (http://www.cdc.gov/nccdphp/dnpa/bmi/calc-bmi.htm or http://www.nhlbisupport.com/bmi/bmicalc.htm). The BMI allows us to compare patients of different heights and weights by giving us a value that takes these differences into account. When a patient's BMI exceeds 35, safety risks increase for both the patient and caregiver. When the BMI exceeds 45, a comprehensive care plan is essential for safety.
- *Weight distribution:* Weight distribution can dramatically affect risk exposure. For instance, if a patient's weight distribution is predominantly around the abdomen, the care plan would look different than if a patient had his/her weight distribution focused around their lower extremities (Dionne, 2002). Weight

distribution also impacts the type of equipment that is most appropriate. A patient with weight concentrations in a certain part of his/her body will more likely need to have a wider bed, chair, and wheelchair. Body shape can also drive, which sling is most appropriate.

- *Cognition:* Regardless of weight, a patient's cognitive status can greatly affect their ability to assist in care such as mobilizing and turning (Hahler, 2002). If a bariatric patient does not have the cognitive capacity to assist during an intervention such as turning, this would change the approach and equipment that the healthcare provider would use.

- *Ability to bear weight:* Upon admission this ought to be one of the first assessments that is made. Bariatric patients who are non-weight bearing expose healthcare professionals to high levels of risk if the patient loses balance or leans on the healthcare provider (Hahler, 2002). This can be avoided if the correct transfer equipment is available. Assessment should be based on the patient's history and an onsite assessment (Dionne, 2002; Hahler, 2002). It is important to assess if falls have occurred prior to admission to the healthcare facility. If the patient has limited ability to bear weight, a physical therapist or rehabilitation physician needs to be involved when developing a mobilization plan. When ordering assistive equipment, an accurate assessment is needed as having too much equipment in the patient area can lead to staff injuries as well due to the inability to position oneself correctly.

- *Pain levels:* Frequently bariatric patients suffer from some form of pain. In many cases this pain is musculoskeletal in nature, such as back pain or joint pains. This pain can affect the mobility of the patient and also the patient's ability to assist in care, such as turning or mobilizing. When a care activity is interrupted due to pain (e.g., the patient cannot continue to turn and has to turn back to his original position), the healthcare provider has an increased level of injury exposure. Having a clear pain assessment is essential for planning further care and determining appropriate equipment.

- *Endurance:* Decreased endurance is commonly observed in bariatric patients (Twedell, 2003). This can lead to a patient needing to sit unexpectedly and, in some cases, can lead to falls. In either circumstance the healthcare provider is exposed to a high level of injury potential. At times the patient's perspective of his ability to mobilize and endure differs from what the healthcare provider observes while offering care. In many cases this can be explained, because the patient has not been mobile to the same extent as at home. Bariatric patients' endurance can drastically decrease even in a few days of bedrest in the hospital. Thus, an actual assessment, in addition to the patient's perspective, is needed to ensure an accurate assessment.

- *Respiratory status:* Most bariatric patients have some level of respiratory impairment (Twedell, 2003). In most cases this is shortness of breath when mobilizing, yet with some patients it is an actual or perceived inability to breathe in certain positions. This can be highly anxiety provoking for patients and lead to unexpected movement or repositioning. Certain equipment (e.g., slings) might lead to the patient experiencing this as well. Thus, an assessment needs to be based on the patient's narrative, as well as a physical assessment while performing certain care components (e.g., mobilization, transfer in a lift). This assessment needs to be performed with the utmost care and with sufficient staff at hand to assist.

- *Complexity of injury exposure:* The authors of this chapter have frequently received the request for a tool that can be easily completed to help identify the level of risk and the level of care needed. As of now, no tool has been shown to capture the complexity of taking care of bariatric patients. Risk levels cannot be calculated simply by adding the different areas of assessment. It is an assessment of the whole situation that will offer the most accurate picture. For instance, if a patient has a BMI of 32, yet has a high level of pain, this can lead to high levels of injury exposure, Whereas a patient with a BMI of 50, who is completely mobile and experiences no pain, can be a much lower source of injury exposure to healthcare professionals. The only way to obtain an accurate risk assessment is to have a professional healthcare provider, trained and experienced in working with bariatric patients (Twedell, 2003). This can be a physician, nurse, clinical nurse specialist (CNS), physical therapist, or other healthcare provider who has received medical training. As of now there is no formalized training offered to teach these skills; thus, much of this knowledge will need to be obtained within one's organization or at national conferences that focus on safe patient handling.

Bariatric Care as Care Specialty

Many hospitals are reluctant to admit medical bariatric patients. There are multiple reasons for this including the need for increased staffing, high-injury potential, and frequent problems with discharge planning (Holland, Krulish, Reich, & Roche, 2001). This population can be very satisfying to work with when staff is supported in providing a care plan driven to promote both patient and staff safety and staff is knowledgeable and has access to equipment that they need to take care of bariatric patients. In several organizations, such as the Mayo Clinic in Rochester and the Veterans Administration in Tampa, staff have accepted the challenge of caring for these patients safely while assuring dignified care. This model of having a certain group of healthcare professionals become experts does not have to be limited to inpatient hospitals. It can be used in alternate settings such as clinics, emergency rooms, or long-term care facilities.

Room Setup

"Get the big boy bed!" was frequently heard in the past when a care unit got word that a bariatric patient was being admitted. In many care facilities the "big boy bed" consisted of two regular size beds bolted together, in others it was an internally constructed bed. These "old fashioned" approaches were unsafe and compromised patient dignity. One of the main concerns was that the patient's condition, other than the weight, was not taken into consideration. In many cases this led to large numbers of staff injuries, especially when the bed was much too large. Caregivers would move excessive distances for patient access and, at times, would have to climb on the bed in order to perform necessary patient handling tasks. These awkward positions increased occupational risk.

Bed Size.   When assessing, which bed is most appropriate, several issues need to be taken into consideration. Body shape or weight distribution influences the most appropriate width of the bed (Holland et al., 2001). In many cases a regular hospital bed can be used. Be aware of bed names that allude to bariatrics. These beds are usually targeted for a certain bariatric population and might not be appropriate for every bariatric patient. Some new bariatric beds are actually expandable offering many options for widths and the added benefit of being able to constrict the width to get through the door. In cases in which a regular hospital bed does not suffice, having a regular but wider bed is a viable option. Other considerations such as the patient's ability to turn independently, level of consciousness, etc. will impact the bed choice. In several hospitals an effective method for obtaining the right bed is to have a CNS with specialized training involved to help with these decisions.

The C or EC Coding System.   Awareness of weight limits on equipment is an ongoing challenge (Holland et al., 2001). There is no industry standard that helps healthcare providers identify what the weight limits are. Using equipment that is not built for the task at hand can dramatically increase the risk of injury for both the patient and the healthcare provider. Having equipment that is too large can also offer increased injury exposure. What should happen in each organization is that all equipment should be coded with weight limits. That can be done by stenciling a code on each piece of equipment. For instance the back of a wheelchair could have C 300 stenciled on it, indicating that the weight capacity is 300 lbs. If coding each piece of equipment is prohibitive, coding all equipment that is larger than the standard with an expanded capacity (EC) code is recommended. Putting verbiage on equipment such as "do not exceed 500 pounds" or "weight limit 500 pounds" is discouraged, as it may be perceived as being offensive or embarrassing to the bariatric patient.

Friction-Reducing Devices.   As a standard part of the room setup a friction-reducing device should be ordered. These devices decrease the amount of strain needed to transfer a patient horizontally (Gallagher, 2000). In most cases less staff is needed to transfer a patient when these devices are used appropriately. When these devices are used consistently and correctly, the number of injuries can be reduced drastically if not eliminated altogether. Having immediate and convenient access to this equipment aids in higher levels of usage, thus decreasing injuries. Many vendors who make friction-reducing devices are now offering them for bariatric populations. Friction-reducing devices can also be used to assist healthcare providers move bariatric patients up in bed. If a device is available that can be kept under the patient while in bed, it decreases turning and the risk exposure associated with placing the device. Yet, unfortunately most products have a deleterious affect on skin integrity with prolonged exposure.

Lifts.   Having the correct "expanded capacity" patient lift along with staff that knows how to use it is a key component to safe care of the bariatric patient (Gallagher, 2000; Meittunen, Snydar, & Meyer, 2001). Taking ample time to introduce a patient and staff to the selected bariatric lift will increase staff adherence and patient acceptance. A common myth is that having received an inservice on a particular lift results in competency for all types of patients. Especially in bariatric patients, adapting how the equipment is used (e.g., correct placement of the sling) can differ from patient to patient. Lifts can also be modified to lift a limb if the patient cannot do that independently. This may be needed for wound care or when performing personal care.

Chairs.   In many cases keeping the bariatric patient mobile is of the greatest importance. Having an EC chair that will accommodate the patient needs to be part of the basic room setup. It is not uncommon to see family members of bariatric patients having the need of larger chairs. Thus, if possible having more than one chair available is highly recommended. Finding the right chair can be challenging. To prevent strain on the healthcare givers back, having a higher chair is recommended. Yet, with shorter patients it might pose safety issues. Ideally the chair ought to be as high as possible, but allow the patient to have his feet touch the ground. The use of footstools should be avoided as it can increase the injury exposure while mobilizing.

Toilets and Commodes.   The typical porcelain toilet has a weight capacity of around 350 pounds. This means that the porcelain can shatter if the weight limit is broken. The practice of placing a block under wall-hung toilets should be avoided. Doing this may prevent the toilet from being pulled out of the wall, but it does not increase the weight capacity of the porcelain and gives a false level of security. When higher weight limits are needed, healthcare facilities can install steel toilets, or the use of portable bariatric commodes (that can frequently be placed over the toilet) can be considered. For the selection of commodes the same criteria as the selection of chairs should be used. Obtain a commode that is as high as possible, yet allow the patients to have their feet touch the ground.

Shower Bars.   Most shower and safety bars also have weight limitations. Having a bariatric patient depend on these shower bars can be dangerous. It is also possible to increase the weight limit by reinforcing the bars, yet for this the walls need to be replaced in most cases. If the shower bars do not accommodate the patient's weight, consider alternatives, for example, the use of a walker or shower chair.

Gowns and Linen.   Obtaining the right-size linen and gowns is an essential part of offering safe care. Having linen the wrong size and not staying in place increases the need of the healthcare provider to turn and tug the patient. This is also true for the right-size gown. Having a gown that is too small not only is uncomfortable and undignified for the patient but also increases the risk of skin tears and pressure ulcers. Furthermore, if a gown is oversized, this can cause the patient to get entangled with resultant tugging and pulling for comfort and safety.

When ordering a specialty bed, a plan needs to be established as to who and how the linen will be supplied that fits that particular bed. It is often the "off" shifts that get exposed to increased risk levels as they are forced to use the wrong-size sheets and gowns as they cannot be procured during their working hours.

The First 48 hours.   The first 48 hours after admission are a key time to set up a plan that will allow for a safe admission (Holland et al., 2001). Ideally an RN should get freed up to develop a care plan and procure supplies and equipment that will be needed. Doing this in addition to a regular patient assignment is usually not feasible. Key components of this first period after admission are:

- *Developing a care plan (mobilization plan):* Many bariatric patients can lose their ability to mobilize or perform self-care activities in only a few days if they do not retain mobility (Hahler, 2002). After mobility has been lost, it can take weeks or even months to get back to baseline. Having a mobility plan that starts as soon as possible can prevent decrease in mobility from occurring. The admitting nurse should develop a mobility plan in collaboration with the physician and physical therapist upon admission. If the patient has restrictions, the plan should be focused on maintaining his baseline mobility within the given restrictions, yet having the plan be something that patient can live with (Gallagher, 1999).
- *Multi-disciplinary meeting:* Each high-risk bariatric patient benefits from a multi-disciplinary meeting shortly after admission to discuss the treatment, care, and discharge planning (de Ruiter, Meittunen, & Sauder, 2001). This meeting should be scheduled as early in the patient's admission. The admitting nurse should schedule a meeting and notify all the stakeholders regarding it.
- *Staffing plan:* Continuity of care providers promotes consistency in how certain procedures, such as using equipment, are performed. In high-risk bariatric patients assessing the work schedule and planning who will take care of the patient ahead of time can decrease the exposure to injury. This also facilitates targeting education of the care plan to the right people.
- *Access of algorithms:* For all high-risk procedures a standard should be established. Algorithms such as described in the "Ergonomic Resource Guide" developed by the VA Patient Safety Center in Tampa, FL should be used (Nelson, 2001 [rev. 2005]). These algorithms have been shown to be beneficial and are

available free of cost on the Internet. Below is an example of a bariatric algorithm that can be used to help a healthcare provider perform safe care is shown in Chapter 5.

- *Obtaining specialty supplies and equipment:* Procuring the correct material and equipment can be time-consuming (Gallagher, 2000). But having the right equipment available is crucial to decreasing injuries. Having equipment ordered and set up in a timely manner should occur within the first 8 h of the admission.
- *Multi-disciplinary meeting:* In the paragraph above, mention has been made about having a multi-disciplinary meeting as early as possible within the admission. All stakeholders should be involved. Here is a listing of possible participants and how their role pertains to the care of the bariatric patients (de Ruiter et al., 2001; Holland et al., 2001).
  - *Nursing*—The primary caregiver of cares to the patient. Nursing is usually also the discipline most affected and impacted by injuries.
  - *Home care*—Can offer insights into levels of mobility prior to admission, as the patient's perspective and healthcare provider's assessment sometimes vary. For example a patient might state "I could get around at home without the use of any aids," yet the homecare nurse's assessment could have been " because the patient was able to hold onto counters and table while getting around his house no additional aids were used." This difference in assessment can lead to different outcome goals.
  - *Physicians*—Have the best overview of the patient history and how long it will take to resolve the issues that lead to the admittance to the healthcare facility. The physician can also write orders as needed during the meeting. If a physician does not attend this initial care conference, this negatively affects the efficacy of the meeting.
  - *Units support coordinator*—This person's role within the organization is to purchase/lease equipment and supplies. The Unit support coordinator usually is well informed about equipment and supply options and how they can be obtained.
  - *Patient and family*—Involving the patient and their family can offer useful information in the barriers experienced in the home setting. Involving the patient early on and obtaining their support in the care plan will promote a safer work environment because helpful tips on how to provide care that is feasible for the patient can be provided. Additionally, co-morbidity, such as depression, might also be brought up by the patient or his family.

- *Physical and occupational therapists*—The role of physical and occupational therapy is to help and establish a sustainable mobilization and self-care plan. The assessments of these disciplines are crucial to determine feasibility of the plans proposed. Creative strategies to overcome mobilization challenges are a part of the PT and OT specialty areas.
- *Dietician*—A common error made when admitting a bariatric patient is that they are instantly placed on a low calorie diet. This can increase the injury exposure when a patient does not have sufficient caloric intake, leading to lethargy and decreased ability to assist in cares and mobilization. It is essential that the patient maintain a nutritional intake that allows them to assist to the maximum of their ability. In some cases the caloric expenditure of a patient at rest might be as high as 2500 cal or more.
- *Safety officer*—Traditionally the safety officers have not been involved in proactive injury prevention. Having the institutional safety officer be a part of the meeting can help increase the understanding of barriers that healthcare providers experience. Also, many safety officers have a strong knowledge base in the area or ergonomics. This knowledge can be tapped to develop new and novel approaches to high-risk procedures. Having the safety office observe the high-risk tasks can be a highly effective way to come up with new strategies. The use of video cameras to analyze high-risk procedures should also be considered.
- *Social work*—As discharge planning is a central part of the multi-disciplinary meeting, social work should be involved from the start. Finding a long-term care facility, if indicated, can be very difficult for this patient population and the more time available to look at options can lead to a successful and timely dismissal. At times the patient will have special equipment needs when going back home; this too frequently leads to the social worker needing ample time.
- *Management/administration*—The best way to get administrative support to purchase or lease specialty equipment is to have them be a part of the meeting. This will give them in-depth insight into the importance and how the procurement of equipment can actually save money by preventing injuries.
- *Others*—On a patient-to-patient basis it should be assessed who should be attending this meeting. Other disciplines could include chaplancy, mental health practitioners, etc. depending on the individual circumstances. In one hospital, pet therapy was even used to help the bariatric patient, who had great

problems mobilizing, feel there was a worthwhile incentive to go through the discomfort of getting up.

- *Meeting format:* Ideally the meeting ought to include meeting time as a team in a conference room and time at the bedside of the patient. As these meetings can be large, it is not advisable to have the whole team go to the bedside. The bedside component of the meeting will include not only discussions with the patient but also assessment of high-risks tasks for which no satisfactory care solutions have been found. It is rare that no solutions are found for high-risk tasks when this multi-disciplinary approach is used.
- The agenda in the sit-down part of the meetings should include the following components (de Ruiter et al., 2001):
  - *History*—including care barriers in the past
  - *Goal of the admission*—In many cases this is the treatment of an acute condition (e.g., cellulites or a pulmonary embolus), yet admissions can easily get extended because this focus is lost during the admission
  - *Mobilization goals/plans*—Focus ought to prevent deterioration of mobility
  - *Barriers*—Such as mental status, family issues, etc.
  - *Discharge plan*—Establish a clear discharge goal. This will assist in keeping focus to the admission. Every unnecessary day in a healthcare facility exposes staff to a high level of injury potential that could have been prevented.

- Ongoing meetings should be determined at the multi-disciplinary meeting or 24 h before the anticipated discharge date.

COMBATIVE PATIENTS

Violence is a significant problem in the society. In the United States, workers encounter approximately 25 million acts of violence annually (Bureau of Justice, 2005). This can include verbal abuse, threats to one's physical safety, or actual physical violence. In 2003, 118 healthcare providers in the United States were murdered while working in their position (US Labor Department, 2004). In healthcare this type of violence is a common occurrence, especially with healthcare providers who work in the frontline in the capacity of direct care providers.

There are two predominate types of injuries that healthcare providers are at risk of obtaining. These will be described as Type A injuries and Type B injuries. Type A injuries result from direct assaults such as bites, scratches, pinches, hits, hair pulling, and more. Unfortunately, most healthcare providers who have given bedside care have experienced one or more of these injuries as part of their practice. Due to the frequency of these occurrence and magnitude of these injuries, many of them go unreported and thus getting accurate statistics is challenging.

Type B injuries, which is the focus of this chapter, are injuries that occur as a result of healthcare providers trying to avoid Type A injuries. The Type B injuries include strains, sprains, herniated disks, and a variety of other injuries that occur as a result of trying to avoid a patient's hit, trying to free one's self when a patient is pulling one's hair, etc. These types of injuries are often not as acute as Type A injuries, but their effect is much longer lasting.

Proposed Solution

For safety purposes it has been shown that utilizing a standardized approach is beneficial, or as the Pennsylvania Patient Safety Collaborative (2001, p. 7) states "Prevention of future errors requires changing systems, not attempting to change individuals." For instance RACE (Relocate, Activate, Contain, Evacuate) is used in most healthcare institutions to help educate staff to respond in case of a fire. Also, if one asks any random person what to do when one catches on fire, one can expect the response "Stop, Drop, and Roll." Yet, when it comes to violent patients, there is no standardized approach even though this is a much more frequent occurrence in healthcare than fires. The concept of standardization as an approach to safety has been used in multiple industries (Hagan, 2001). This is especially true of aviation where prior to each flight the pilots go through a pre-determined checklist to ensure safety. Pilots also have been trained to respond to emergent situations in a standardized manner (Hawkins & Orlady, 1993; Wells, & Rodriquez, 2004). Healthcare has lacked a standardized approach to preventing both Type A and B injuries as a result of patient and/or family aggression. The following model offers a structure in which healthcare teams can be trained to offer a standardized approach to dealing with violence and aggression in healthcare.

The ROAD (Relocate, Organize, Assign, and De-escalate) approach has been developed, after analyzing multiple patient escalations, to give healthcare providers a tool to safely deal with aggression in their work environment. It is a standardized approach that can offer healthcare providers guidance to handling acute behavioral outbursts. Depending on institutional policies, it might need to be modified not only to ensure staff and patient safety but also to comply with institutional policies.

Relocate.   The first step is realizing that each healthcare provider has a role in preventing injury to him/herself. Historically, healthcare providers have put themselves in harm's way to protect patients, even when the harm toward themselves could have been avoided without a negative outcome to the patient. Thanks to the efforts by nursing organizations in Europe, the United States and Australia, this approach is changing. The American Nurses Association has reaffirmed this as they inserted the 5th Standard, which states that nurses have the same responsibility toward self as toward the patients (American Nurses Association, 2001). When situations occur in which a patient or family is trying to harm a healthcare provider, the provider should remove him/herself from the situation as soon as possible. If this is not taught and reinforced to healthcare providers, it is not usually a natural response. When a crisis occurs, it is not the ideal time to review what the most ideal response would be, nor to review the code of ethics. Removing oneself from a dangerous patient/family encounter needs to become an automatic, standardized approach.

Organize.   The next step is to organize staff in a code-like manner. Depending on organizational policy, security might need to be called. It is advisable to remove staff not trained in the ROAD method. Another action is to remove anyone not a part of the professional team in the work area such as visitors, consulting teams, and students. Unfortunately, escalation often attracts people who ought not be involved. The size of the intervention team depends on the type of violence one is dealing with. It is important to have enough staff available to regain control over the situation. Having too many staff members can increase the exposure to musculoskeletal injuries when an intervention is needed. This because it is harder to assume proper body mechanics when one lacks the space to position oneself.

Assign.   The third step is to assign two people to coordinate the intervention. One person should be coordinating the situation outside of the room where this escalation is occurring and one person should be in charge inside the room where the escalation has occurred. The person outside the room should be assigned based on their ability to coordinate and delegate staff; often a person with a directive style can be very effective at this. They can keep people away from the area who do not have to be there and also prevent staff from barging into the situation trying to "save the day." The person who is in charge of the situation inside the room is ideally a person who has a good report with the person who has escalated, or has strong interpersonal skills. They should be able to stay calm (or at least appear calm) even if they are verbally being attacked. If either of the people assigned does not possess the appropriate skills, this can drastically increase the injury risk to all involved in the situation.

De-Escalate. De-escalation should always be the goal of a situation. There are numerous courses and techniques that discuss de-escalation techniques. An example is the PIP method that has shown much effectiveness in mental health settings. Each setting should have a plan what to do if de-escalation fails. In some organizations it might be security that takes over, and in others healthcare providers might be trained. Even though training does not eliminate the injury potential, it can decrease it dramatically. This is true especially for musculoskeletal injuries (Type 2 injuries). Training staff during annual competencies in a concept such as ROAD should be considered in each healthcare organization. Having all staff prepared what to do when a patient or family escalates is an important step in injury prevention.

Use of the ROAD approach can prevent staff injuries. There is, however, a tendency to underestimate the potential for combative behaviors. Being caught unaware increases risk for injury to both the caregiver and the patient. When implementing the patient handling algorithms (Chapter 5; Nelson, 2001 [rev. 2005]), an extra staff member should always be present if the patient has a history of combative or unpredictable behaviors.

COGNITIVE IMPAIRMENTS

Cognitively impaired patients have difficulty following instructions, are likely to resist care, and may exhibit combative behavior (Galski, Palasz, Bruno, & Walker, 1994). The impairment can be acute (e.g., delirium brought on by medications) or chronic, such as patients with such diagnoses as traumatic brain injury, cerebral vascular accident (CVA), mentally retardation, Alzheimer's disease, etc. Even without a past history of physical aggression, one should anticipate the possibility of a combative behaviors given the cognitive limitations.

The MAP Approach

A standardized approach should be implemented to prevent acts of aggression from occurring. A standardized approach, such as the MAP (Minimize, Antecedents, and Plan), can significantly decrease the number of injuries that occur related to the patient actions. What healthcare givers often consider unpredictable actions of violence in cognitively impaired patients can often be predicted and averted.

Minimize

The first step is to decrease stimuli that can exacerbate agitation. Too much noise or action can easily increase a cognitively impaired patient's level of restlessness. Yet in practice, confused patients are often placed close to the nurses' station, with a rationale that they can be better observed. Sound levels can be extremely high around nurses' stations. Noise levels of 80–100 dB during the day and in the low 70s during the night (Lower, Bonsack, & Guion, 2003). These noise levels are comparable to the noise levels found adjacent to a highway. But in contrast to the sounds around a highway the sounds around a nursing station have greater variation in the types of sounds. For example, people laughing, phones ringing, and equipment alarms are just a few illustrations. This variety of sounds can be more agitating to a cognitively impaired patient than monotone noises. Another common practice is to place two people who are cognitively impaired in the same room. This can be advantageous for staffing and budgetary reasons but it can easily agitate patients who often have limited ability to comprehend what is occurring around them. Private rooms are highly encouraged to achieve a quiet environment that has minimal stimuli. In many cognitively impaired patients, television can also work as a stimulant; thus, the use should be used conscientiously. Calm music may be a better alternative. Consideration should also be given to the room lighting. Having fluorescent lights on above the patient can be a source of stimuli. Using a lamp shade or indirect lighting can minimize unwanted stimuli.

Antecedents

When caring for persons with cognitive impairments, we can frequently predict when certain occurrences increase agitation. These antecedents of agitation can include turning, patient transfers, or patient transport. A simple action, such as medication administration or feeding can also be an antecedent. A change in care, such introducing new caregivers, can also lead to increased agitation. What all these situations have in common is that they cause a disruption for the cognitively impaired patient, with resultant agitation or fear. Upon admission these antecedents need to be closely assessed and documented. Having a clear awareness of when injury exposure is increased allows for injury prevention. This will be discussed in the next paragraph.

Plan

Having a comprehensive plan is the key to decreasing injuries in cognitively impaired patients. The plan should include both environmental and care delivery components. Environmentally, the plan should call for an area that has a low level of stimuli. In many facilities this will require somewhat of a culture change as these populations often cared for areas that are highly saturated with a variety of environmental stimuli. The care delivery plan should list the antecedents and describe what actions the healthcare provider should take to avoid agitation or increasing fear levels of this patient population. For instance, if the plan identifies turning the patient as an antecedent, maybe thought should be given to the frequency of turning and also to plan these activities during times that the appropriate staff is available. If bathing is identified as an antecedent, thought should be given regarding, which times of the day the patient is most receptive to this care. This might mean that bathing will occur in the early evening rather than what is traditionally done, in the early part of the morning. Having a primary caregiver or a small group of primary caregivers can help achieve a higher level of consistency and better follow-through of the care plan.

PATIENTS WITH SEVERE PAIN

Handling patients with severe pain requires careful attention. The goals of safe patient handling with this patient population include safety to the patient and the caregiver, as well as minimizing pain. Severe pain in patients can contribute to staff injuries for a variety of reasons. There may be decreased patient cooperation and participation due to anticipated or actual pain. The patient may move unexpectedly due to severe pain or fear. Also, healthcare providers may be distracted due to the patient's expression of pain. Pain is also experienced differently by different individuals (McCaffery & Beebe, 1989). For example, the same surgery on two different people may result in very different responses to pain. Thus, it is important to assess the pain response in each individual and not to generalize.

Movement often causes pain to increase, which frequently evokes a psychological response in both the patient and the caregiver. When the patient anticipates pain with movement, he/she may be less cooperative, requiring the staff to provide more assistance than may be anticipated. In order to avoid pain or in response to pain, patients may move suddenly and unexpectedly, thus putting the healthcare provider at an increased risk of injury. If the patient has repeatedly been moved in a rough manner, an increased fear of moving will make further transfers and patient handling more difficult and met with more resistance. There is also a significant psychological response in the caregiver. Naturally, most people do not want to inflict more pain on someone. To minimize the pain of moving a patient, a caregiver may unfortunately be willing to compromise their own safety and handling techniques to reduce the psychological stress of increasing a patient's pain with movement.

Using a consistent approach in handling patients with pain can minimize their pain as well as their "fear-response" to being moved. A comprehensive plan is needed for pain prevention (McCaffery & Beebe, 1989). It should ideally be a multi-disciplinary approach, using input from those involved in pain management as well as those who will be directly involved in patient handling tasks. The plan should include medication regimes, activities permitted and/or to be encouraged, the scheduling of those activities, as well as the number of people and equipment to be used during patient handling.

Pain levels should be assessed on an ongoing basis with medication regimes based on those assessments. A typical plan to pre-medicate patients half an hour before activities may not be ideal for all patients. The medication regime should be based on ongoing pain assessments. If changes are made in the medication schedule, this needs to be clearly communicated and updated in the comprehensive plan. Adequate pain control with medication prior to patient handling will decrease both the patient's and the caregiver's response to pain, allowing for increased safety for the healthcare provider and increased patient confidence in the care received.

Not only is timing of medication important, but also the timing of activities is critical. The most strenuous activities for the patient should be scheduled during the time of the day when the patient typically has the least pain. For example, if they tend to be more relaxed and in less pain in the afternoon, perhaps their bathing could occur then, rather than first thing in the morning. An activities schedule should also be based on ongoing pain assessments and made part of the comprehensive plan. The number of activities may also need to be limited so as not to overburden the patient.

The comprehensive plan should also include the number of people needed to handle the patient safely. Any equipment and/or special precautions should also be clearly stated in the plan. Based on the patient, a person in severe pain may move easier in one direction or with specific equipment.

In general, using a firm but gentle hand placement with as few adjustments in hand position as possible will help the patient handling go more smoothly. Locate points of control where there is less pain when possible. If a patient has primarily back pain, using both the shoulder and hips as points of control with minimizing as much twisting or bending will generally be the most comfortable way for the patient. If the shoulder or upper extremity is the primary source of pain, supporting the arm gently but firmly while using the mid back and hip as the points of control will make the movement easier. With a lower extremity pain source, supporting the legs and controlling the back and hips will make the movement more comfortable. In addition, using equipment such as abdominal binders or back supports may make patient handling safer in patients with severe abdominal and back pain.

It is also important to coordinate movements both with the patient and with anyone else assisting with patient handling. Counting or some signal for movement is essential to minimize jerking, which can greatly increase pain. One must also be aware not to make too cautious of movements that are insufficient and thus require additional movement. Movements should be made efficiently, assuredly, and with as much precision so that neither inadequate nor excessive movement occurs.

PATIENTS WITH EXTENSIVE WOUNDS

Patients with extensive wounds often have bandages and/or exposed tissue that needs to be protected (Black & Hawks, 2004). Disruption of bandages, shearing forces, and excessive pressure can worsen wounds and prolong healing, making safe patient handling of this population extremely important as well as challenging.

The location/s, size, severity, and type of bandage of the wound/s provide a unique challenge to the caregiver when handling these patients. The challenge is not to compromise one's own safety during patient handling while protecting the wound as much as possible. Typically, these patients also have extreme pain; suggestions under handling patients with pain need to be considered as well.

It is important to be fully aware of what wounds a patient has, their severity, and their locations. The most severe and painful wounds should be given greatest consideration. Make sure bandages are secure and/ or loose bandages are removed if it is time for a dressing change. This will help minimize disruption to the healing process caused by bandage slippage. It also helps protect caregivers by avoiding sudden, impulsive movements to try to resecure bandages during the patient handling process. In addition to bandages, one must also be aware of any tubes or drains common with extensive wounds before beginning the movement.

Adequate exposure precautions need to be taken by all caregivers involved in handling a patient with severe wounds. That includes, at a minimum gloves, and most likely gowns and other protective clothing depending on the wounds. Improperly used protective clothing can compromise a caregiver's safety as well. Loose gowns can become snagged, loose face masks can interfere with vision, and loose gloves can cause slippage. It is important to use well-fitting gloves and secure gowns and masks tightly so that they will not become a hindrance and compromise safety.

Using equipment such as reduced-friction draw sheets, sliding boards, and binders for abdominal wounds can make patient handling and transfers safer for the caregiver and more comfortable for the patient. Hydraulic lifts should be used with considerable care as they can increase sheer and pressure forces on compromised tissue.

PATIENTS WITH NEUROLOGICAL CONDITIONS

Many other patient conditions warrant consideration by the healthcare provider to prevent injuries. To name a few, they include patients with neurological conditions such as multiple sclerosis (MS), CVA, cerebral palsy (CP), and spinal cord injuries (SCI). With each of these there is the common occurrence of spasms with transfers and patient handling. If the healthcare provider is unsuspecting or unprepared for such body spasms during a move, injury can easily occur. The healthcare provider must anticipate spastic movements in patients with many types of neurological conditions and have appropriate equipment and number of staff present for all patient handling. Often keeping patients in a more flexed position may help to diminish spastic reflexes during movement. As well, smooth, solid motions without jerking or sudden movements can help improve the safety with patient handling. The patient may also be able to advise if and when spasms are present and what triggers them.

Another consideration with some patients with certain neurological conditions affecting safe patient handling is their cognitive status. Many have impaired cognitive abilities increasing the risk of injury to the healthcare provider. Particularly, impulsivity and impaired safety awareness in patients can easily cause injuries to the unsuspecting healthcare provider. Clear, concise directions to patients as well as having the appropriate equipment and assistance needed can help to reduce the number of injuries to healthcare providers.

Another patient population for special consideration is that with orthostatic hypotension, where the blood pressure drops when moved into a more upright position. This may occur in patients as a result of prolonged bedrest, post-surgical, a side-effect of some medications, or a complication of some diseases. For example, patients with Parkinson's disease often have problems with orthostatic hypotension. There is also a condition, postural tachycardia syndrome (POTS) disease, where one of the primary symptoms is orthostatic hypotension. Patients who are known to have or are likely to have problems with blood pressure should be moved slowly and in increments into an upright position, frequently assessing for symptoms of orthostatic hypotension. Moving a patient too quickly and without monitoring symptoms may lead to a patient fainting, causing considerable risk to both the healthcare provider and the patient.

Patients who have suffered motor vehicle accidents (MVA) should also be given special consideration with patient handling. Not only do they frequently have multiple injury sights but they are also likely to be in significant pain and may also have problems with orthostatic hypotension. They also may have suffered other problems, which have yet to be fully diagnosed such as a traumatic brain injury, fractures, or soft-tissue injuries. Adequate personnel and equipment for safe patient handling as well as the considerations mentioned earlier in this chapter for pain and orthostatic hypotension should be utilized to decrease injury risks.

PEDIATRIC PATIENTS

Pediatric patients, while generally much lighter in weight, may pose increased safety risks to caregivers. In part, because of their lighter weight, caregivers may underestimate the need for additional help when handling patients of this population. Pediatric patients, especially when in an unfamiliar environment, under medications, and in pain/not feeling well, may have difficulty understanding their situation. As a result, pediatric patients may demonstrate increased fear and resistance to being moved, especially by a stranger. When scared and confused, pediatric patients can exhibit extraordinary force. Children are also less restrained than adults when it comes to hitting, biting, and kicking, especially when forced to do something they do not want to.

Parents/family members, in trying to protect the child, may create an environment of increased anxiety and fear for the child. There are situations where the parents may be overly involved or with poor understanding of the child's condition. They may inadvertently or intentionally interfere with patient handling, thus compromising the caregivers' safety as well as of the patients.

The fortunate thing about children is they do tend to be extremely adaptable. It is important to try to make pediatric patients as comfortable as possible and to understand their situation as well as possible. Using simple words and explanations, prepare patients as much as possible before handling or moving them. It is also helpful to involve family members as well. Parents are also a wealth of information to healthcare providers in helping to understand what escalates their children and what has a calming effect on them. In other situations, depending on the patient's condition and prior experience of the parents, anxious parents may need to be distracted with other tasks or asked to leave to decrease the fear imparted to the patient.

Key elements while handling pediatric elements are to take time to get to know the child. Make sure you are interacting with the child verbally. Call them by name so that they have some sense of familiarity. If you know they have a certain passion such as collecting cards or a sport, ask them about it. If for some reason the relationship between a child and a caregiver does not flow smoothly do not hesitate to make staffing changes. This is not necessarily a negative reflection on the caregiver, as children frequently work much better with certain people.

SUMMARY

Occupational injuries during patient handling tasks remain a critical issue in healthcare delivery. This is especially true in certain patient populations such as the bariatric patient, the confused or combative patient, the patient in extreme pain or with extensive wounds, patients with certain neurological conditions, and pediatric patients. Even though these patient populations require their own unique approaches as described in this chapter, there are commonalities among them to decrease risk exposure. Planning ahead and anticipating problems, using a multi-disciplinary approach, providing continuing care through a care plan, and the utilization of appropriate and/or specialized equipment should provide a foundation to decrease staff injuries.

REFERENCES

Allison, D. B., & Saunders, S. E. (2000). Obesity in North America: an overview. *Medical Clinics of North America, 84*(2), 305–332.

American Nurses Association. (2001). *Code of ethics with interpretive statements*. Washington, DC: Author.

Baptiste, A., Meittunen, E., & Bertschinger, G. (2004). Technology solutions for bariatric populations. *Journal of the Association of Occupational Health Professionals in Healthare, 24*(2), 18–22.

Barr J., & Cunneen, J. (2001). Understanding the bariatric client and providing a safe hospital environment. *Clinical Nurse Specialist, 15*(5), 219–223.

Black, J., Hawks, J., & Keene, A. (2004). *Medical-surgical nursing: Clinical management for positive outcomes*. Philadelphia: W. B. Saunders Co.

Bureau of Justice. (2005). National Crime Victimization Survery. Retrieved April 20, 2005, from www.ojp.usdoj.gov

Centers for Disease Control (CDC). (2002). Obesity still on the rise new data show. Retrieved March 28, 2004, from http://www.cdc.gov/nccdphp/dnpa/press/archive/obesity_10_2002.htm

de Ruiter, H. P., Meittunen, E., & Sauder, K. (2001). Improving safety for caregivers through collaborative practice. *Journal of Healthcare Safety: Compliance and Infection Control, 5*(2), 61–64.

Dionne, M. (2002). One size does not fit all. *Rehab Management: The Interdisciplinary Journal of Rehabilitation*. Retrieved April 21, 2005 from http://www.rehabpub.com/features/32002/1.asp

Dionne, M. (2005). Raising the bar in bariatric care. *PT Magazine, March*, 24–30.

Gallagher, S. (1999). Tailoring care for obese patients. *RN, 62*(5), 43–50.

Gallagher, S. (2000). Rehab products: questions and answers. How do your bariatric products help make transfers easy and safe? *Advance for Directors in Rehabilitation, 9*(3), 71.

Galski, T., Palasz, J., Bruno, R. L., & Walker, J. E. (1994). Predicting physical and verbal aggression on brain traume unit. *Archives of Physical Medicine and Rehabilitation, 75*(4), 280–283.

Hagan, P. (2001). *Accident prevention manual for business and industry: Administration and programs* (12th ed.). Washington, DC: National Safety Council.

Hahler, B. (2002). Morbid obesity: a nursing care challenge. *Dermatology Nursing, 14*(4), 249–256.

Hawkins, F., & Orlady, H. (1993). *Human factors in flight* (2nd ed.). Burlington, VT: Ashgate Publishing.

Holland, D., Krulish, Y., Reich, H., & Roche, J. (2001). How to creatively meet care needs of the morbidly obese. *Nursing Management, 32*(6), 39–41.

Kuczmarski, R., & Flegal, K. (2000). Criteria for definition of overweight in transition: background and recommendations for the United States. *American Journal of Clinical Nutrition, 72*(5), 1074–1081.

Lower, J., Bonsack C., & Guion J. (2003). Piece and quit. *Nursing Management, 34*(4), 40a–40d.

McCaffery, M., & Beebe, A. (1989). *Pain: Clinical manual for nursing practice.* St. Louis, MO: C. V. Mosby.

Meittunen, E., Matzke, K., & Sobczak, S., (1999). Identification of risk factors for a challenging ergonomic issue: the patient transfer. *Journal of Healthcare Safety: Compliance and Infection Control, 3*(1), 9–19.

Meittunen, E., McCormack, H., & Sobczak, S. (2000). Evaluation of patient transfer tasks using multiple data sources. *Journal of Healthcare Safety: Compliand and Infection Control, 4*(1), 13–16.

Meittunen, R., Snydar, B., & Meyer, M. (2001). The process and results of departmental specific surveys for health care organizations: successful program. *American Association of Occupational Health Nurses, 49*(4), 187–193.

Must, A., Spadano, J., Coakley, E. H., Field, A. E., Colditz, G., & Dietz, W. H. (1999). The disease burden associated with overweight and obesity. *Journal of the American Medical Association, 282*(16), 1523–1529.

Nelson, A. L. (Ed.). (2001 [rev. 2005]). *Patient care ergonomics resource guide: Safe patient handling and movement.* Tampa, FL: Veterans Administration Patient Safety Center of Inquiry. Available at: http://www.patientsafetycenter.com/Safe%20Pt%20Handling%20Div.htm

Nelson, A., Lloyd, J., Fragala, G., Matz, M., Amato, M., Bowers, J., Moss-Cureton, S., Ramsey, G., & Lentz, K. (2003). Safe patient handling and movement: preventing back injury among nurses requires careful selection of the safest equipment and techniques. *American Journal of Nursing, 103*(3), 32–43.

Nelson, A., Baptiste, A., de Ruiter, H., Thomason, S., Belwood, J. (in press). Approaches for safe patient handling and movement of bariatric patients. *American Journal of Nursing.*

Pennsylvania Patient Safety Collaborative. (2001). *Elements of a culture of safety: Patient safety is our top priority.* Harrisburg, PA: Author.

Twedell, D. (2003). Physical assessment of the bariatric person. *The Journal of Continuing Education in Nursing, 34*(4), 147–148.

US Labor Department. (2004). News of the US Labor Department. Wednesday, September, 22, 2004.

Wells, A., & Rodriquez, C. (2004). *Commercial aviation safety* (4th ed.). New York: McGraw-Hill Professional.

Youngkin, E. Q., & Kissinger, J. F. (1999). Obesity. In E. Q. Youngkin, K. J. Sawin, J. F. Kissinger, & D. S. Israel (Eds.), *Pharmacotherapeutics: A primary care clinical guide* (pp. 731–746). Stamford, CT: Appleton & Lange.

CHAPTER TWELVE

Physical Environment for Provision of Nursing Care:

Design for Safe Patient Handling

Jocelyn Villeneuve ASSTSAS*

There is clear evidence that the vast majority of occupational injuries involving caregivers are directly related to patient transfers (Owen, 2004; Stubbs, Buckle, Hudson, & Rivers, 1983). In patient care units, most caregiver injuries occur in patients' rooms and bathrooms. This chapter proposes some criteria for designing healthcare environments based on ergonomics.

ERGONOMIC APPROACH

The ergonomic approach is based on a systemic view of work situations, as well as observations and measurements in the field which, combined with scientific knowledge, can be used to propose modifications that are beneficial to everyone. An improvement in the caregiver's work environment is likely to have a positive impact on patient comfort and mobility.

*ASSTSAS is a non-profit joint organization dedicated to health and safety prevention for healthcare workers in Quebec, Canada. (Association paritaire pour la santé et la sécurité du travail, secteur affaires Sociales); www.asstsas.qc.ca

To make patient transfer tasks safer, several elements must be considered: how the work is organized (teams, schedules, etc.), the condition of the patient and of the caregiver, staff training, available equipment, and layout of the premises. To successfully prevent and reduce occupational injuries, action must be taken on all of these fronts simultaneously.

This chapter focuses mainly on workplace design. As early as ASSTSAS symposium (ASSTSAS, 1992), we presented a full-scale model of an "ergonomic patient room." An ergonomic room is a place where a patient can have a comfortable stay and caregivers can provide the necessary care without a risk of injury. This assumes that the technical aids and equipment used for this purpose are available, and that there is enough room to use them properly.

USER CONSULTATION

The success of a construction or renovation project is based in part on dialog with direct users, particularly nursing staff. It is important to intervene effectively right from the preliminary design stage of an architectural project, preferably at the planning stage, when the surfaces to be built or renovated are defined (Villeneuve, 2000, 2004).

A "committee of experts," comprising RNs, LPNs, CNAs, occupational therapists, physiotherapists, and a nurse manager, should be convened to examine risks associated with patient care. The committee must obtain a clear mandate from management and the project manager. Its recommendations can then be submitted to the architects who produce the preliminary drafts for the design. The committee should have decision-making power over the final versions of the plans.

The committee should compile an overview of the problems associated with patient transfers through a variety of means, that is, analysis of occupational injuries and identification of corrective measures to be taken in the new facilities, current and future clients, as well departments that require heavy transfers.

One way to proceed is with a step-by-step analysis of the flow of typical patients from the entrance to the exit of the building. During this process, it is important to identify the specific locations where handling is done and to make provisions for the most appropriate equipment for eliminating as much manual handling as possible.

In a large architectural project, users' committees should be formed by department or by theme, and must be composed of representatives of the executives and workers concerned by the project. Their mandate is to help define requirements and then provide an informed opinion on the design proposals, based on their expertise in the field.

Conditions for Staff Participation

The most important conditions are commitment and consistent support from upper management. The project manager should be skilled at participatory management and take a similar approach. Listening to users' needs and respecting the professional prerogatives of the various people involved in the project should be central objectives. The following conditions should therefore be met by hospital management, design professionals (architects, engineers, etc.), employees, and their trade union representatives.

For Hospital Management. Transparency and sharing of information are essential conditions with the exception, of course, of certain information that must remain confidential.

An atmosphere of trust can develop quickly, and numerous experiences have shown that demands by workers and department heads are realistic and do not necessarily increase the costs of a project. As one hospital manager pointed out, *"The employees didn't make any frivolous demands. On the contrary, all of the proposals submitted were relevant and some were major."*

The transition and start-up of the new facility is much easier if staff has been involved right from the beginning of the project, particularly when work organization technologies and staffing are changed.

There is generally no budget overrun or scheduling delay when the process is initiated from the very start of the project. On the contrary, considerable savings can be achieved by significantly reducing modifications that must be made after the construction work has been completed.

For Designers, Architects, and Engineers. Availability and openness to comments from the staff are essential. Professionals should also be skilled at providing simple explanations to technical questions and managing demands that may not always be consistent. The project manager has to play the role of intermediary between the designers and staff who work on the floor.

It sometimes happens, in fact, that different groups make contrary requests. Professionals' skill at interpreting these requests and negotiating creative compromises is therefore crucial. On the other hand, they are not always well informed about the impact the project will have on the social dynamics of the institution.

Professionals usually have trouble accepting last-minute interventions once they are at the final preliminary or detailed planning stage, and rightly so, because any significant change means revising their plans. Often, additional fees are also charged. It is therefore the responsibility of the institution to initiate the consultation process right from the start of the project, to avoid this type of inconvenience.

As for Employees and Trade Union Representatives.   They are willing to participate as long as their opinions and comments are listened to. That is why it is very important to clearly define the mandate and powers of joint committees (employees and management) from the outset. These committees usually only have recommending power, which can be real power if management takes the process seriously. Hence, the importance of following up proposed recommendations and explaining why some of them were not chosen or were modified.

Giving staff time off with pay or time off in lieu should be included in the budget to avoid creating overwork for those who remain on duty.

DYNAMIC SIMULATIONS

Simulations should be organized for the most common patient transfer locations: patients' rooms and bathrooms. Real size simulation is the best way to validate the functionality of these strategic locations and to prevent occupational injuries. The simulations must be performed by actual users, but of course the patient's role can be played by an employee.

Systematic simulation exercises performed in typical patient transfer locations always result in significant changes being made to the architectural plans. It is very difficult to anticipate everything from a plan, particularly for people who are not accustomed to working with them. Simulations in real-life situations provide a much more realistic view, and can accurately anticipate future tasks and prevent errors or omissions. This type of exercise is very economical and extremely profitable. For instance, when we were involved in a new hospital construction project, we were able to conduct this simulation in all of the typical rooms within 4 days. This had a major impact, not only on room configuration but also on the exterior shape of the building. It is very important to invite architects to take part in these simulations. This allows them to better understand the caregivers and patients safety needs, and thus respond to them to the best of their abilities.

Methodology

The *dynamic simulation procedure* can be applied to all steps of the design phase—programming, design draft, preliminary plans and specifications, and detailed plans and specifications. It can also be reproduced at the three functional analysis levels—in other words, at the level of the whole building (macroscopic), the various departments (mesoscopic), and the individual workstations (microscopic). The logic of this simulation method is to start by choosing priority future scenarios, for instance, related to patient transfers. The idea is to place real users in a mock-up of a design concept and simulate the scenarios. The suitability of the design concept and the scenarios can then be diagnosed. This leads to proposals for changes in the design concept or the scenarios, and finally to a design that fully satisfies user expectations (see Figure 12.1).

Simulation also provides an opportunity to confront different viewpoints in a positive way. Architects, engineers, department heads, employees, and ergonomists may have very different views of the work. This diversity of viewpoints is not an obstacle to project development. On the contrary, it provides an overall vision of the projected situation without which the design exercise may be defective. Simulation is thus an excellent way to confront different viewpoints and thus reach a creative compromise.

Simulation Props

The major props used to create dynamic future activity simulations are *the enlarged plan, three-dimensional (3-D) representations, full-scale simulation with mock-up*, and *prototype*.

Any of these simulation props can be used, depending on the circumstances. All simulations begin with a plan. However, users may not be used to reading design plans, and their natural ability to do so may vary tremendously. In fact, the majority find this task difficult, especially when the plan is on a small scale. For this reason, inexperienced users must have guidance to help them read and interpret the plan. It is also better to work with larger scale plans (1:50 rather than 1:100).

3-D simulation props are much better at providing users with a meaningful representation. The closer the simulation is to reality, the better the results will be in terms of the reliability of the design.

3-D simulation software is now available at a reasonable cost. On request, architectural firms can easily provide 3-D representations produced with AutoCad that are tremendously useful for visualizing the building as a whole or specific areas inside the building.

One excellent type of simulation is the full-scale simulation because it has the advantage of involving real users in action. It is relatively simple to organize, either in comparable existing facilities or in a room that is large enough to reproduce the situation with a mock-up of all fixed and movable equipment (see Figure 12.2).

Simulations such as this are appropriate when copies of the same layout model will be reproduced a number of times in the building. This is often the case in hospitals, where the different floors follow

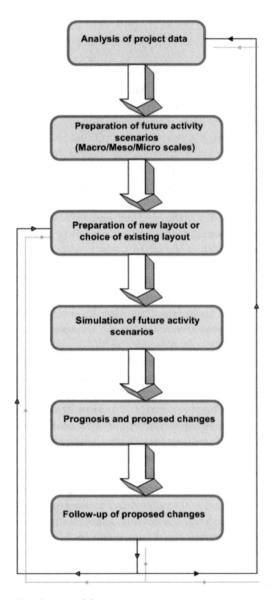

FIGURE 12.1   Simulation of future activities.

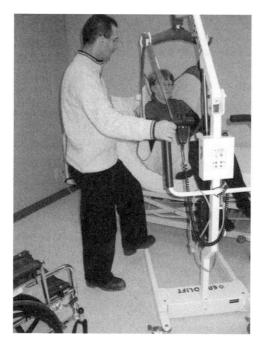

FIGURE 12.2   Simulation with mock-up of typical patient room.

the same pattern. They are also appropriate for testing operations of a critical nature, where errors may have serious human or financial consequences.

It is sometimes necessary to use prototypes to validate anthropomorphic dimensions and the functioning of certain expensive installations before making a final decision on design.

Simulation Follow-Up.   Once a simulation has been completed, the people involved are in a position to decide whether or not the design concept is appropriate for the work context as defined. This is known as the prognosis.

The prognosis can take three directions:

- The design concept works well in the context defined by the scenario
- The design concept does not work well and has to be reviewed in whole or in part (modified design concept)
- The design concept would work in a different context (modified scenario)

The design concept must be adapted to the future activity scenario, and not vice versa. In an architectural project involving substantial sums of money, users have a right to expect that the layout will meet their expectations. The design must satisfy users' needs, instead of trying to change working methods to suit the proposed design concept. This is not always easy, and creative compromise is often required, especially in renovation projects where additional constraints are imposed by the existing building.

The results of the simulation must be written up, and rigorous follow-up is required to define new measures until a satisfactory solution can be found, in terms of operational functioning and the health, safety, and comfort of users.

VISITS TO REFERENCE SITES

Visits to reference sites are an excellent way of creating a more open attitude to new operating methods and new approaches that are often derived from new technology. Such visits encourage those involved to think about changes in practice and move away from what presently exists. They are therefore a vital component in the project definition process. They tend to be organized spontaneously, but all too often they are improvised and achieve only part of their goal (Zimring, 1997).

Here are some of the basic conditions required to ensure that visits to reference sites are as useful as possible.

Forming the Project Group

Whatever the type of visit, the project group should include a decision-maker, the project manager, direct user representatives, a workplace health and safety representative, and the professionals involved. Each person has a different viewpoint and the questions he or she raises will help the group understand how the site works, how it is organized, and how all this is relevant to their own project.

Establishing Objectives

Wherever possible, the project group should meet beforehand to prepare the visit and establish precise objectives. What specific aspects does the group wish to consider? What information is needed on operations, care approaches, technologies, layout designs, and ergonomic, health, and safety questions?

The group members should draw up questions in advance, although there should, of course, be room for spontaneous questions that arise during the visit. There is nothing to prevent the questions from being sent to the site beforehand. This will allow the host team to prepare for the visit and obtain copies of any relevant documentation.

Selecting Sites

Preference should be given to sites that meet the project's general objectives. It is best to visit newly constructed or newly renovated buildings because the technologies and layouts will reflect recent changes in the medical field. Other sites may be chosen because they are of more specific interest in that they contain interesting workstations, room layouts, equipment, or furniture.

The number of sites visited will depend on the complexity of the project and the expertise available within the group. Sometimes new functions may be added, with which users do not have much experience. In such cases, it is essential to make several site visits, so that users are able to give clear opinions on the department's future orientations and on the layout proposals submitted by the architects.

Informing the Host Team of the Visitors' Expectations

The host team should be told about the visiting group's expectations, so that it can ensure that the right people are available. Indeed, the choice of interlocutors is very important. "Tourist" type visits, led by the institution's public relations officer, should be avoided, since they will give a very superficial idea of the premises and the positive aspects of the building. It is just as important to know the negative aspects, and it is therefore important to meet the people who are most familiar with operations. The local renovation or construction project manager should also be present.

During the Visit

An introduction to the department and the background to the project should normally precede the site visit. The classical way of conducting a visit is to follow the chronological order of the department's operations, beginning, for example, with the patient arriving in the waiting room and moving through the various stages up to discharge from the hospital. At each stage, the group should be free to ask questions.

The following are some examples of key questions that might be asked:

- What are the department's main goals and preferred approach?
- How many professional and managerial staff work on each shift?
- What is the client profile?
- What is the volume of activities, and are there any seasonal or other variations (evening, night, weekend)?
- What are the main routes—patients, visitors, staff, clean, and dirty supplies?
- What are the main types of workplace injuries that occur?
- What technologies are used? Why were these particular technologies selected? What are their advantages and disadvantages, costs, and benefits? How reliable are they? How much maintenance do they need?
- What is the logic of the layout design selected? Why was this particular architectural design selected?
- What works well? What are they proudest of?
- What would they improve if they could start over?

It is essential to document the visit, by taking notes, photos or a video, as needed. The premises and equipment should also be measured if necessary, and group members should ask questions about the suppliers, the quality of after-sales service, and the advantages and disadvantages of the products, equipment, and furniture.

It is best to hold a group meeting immediately after the visit, so that members can identify the elements worth keeping and those that should be rejected, while their memories are fresh.

Producing a Report

It is essential to produce a report on the visit. One person should be assigned specifically to this task, and his or her role is to gather the information collected by the group members. A preliminary report should be sent to the members for comments and additions. A final version, illustrated with photos, can then be prepared, emphasizing the aspects to be used in the project. The report is then kept in the project file.

ZERO LIFT

The most promising approach for preventing back injuries in health care would be to eliminate manual lifting, by making maximum use of mechanical aids. Training programs on safe lifting techniques do not give good results without modifying the working environment and providing the proper equipment (St. Vincent, Lortie, & Tellier, 1987). Dealing with this issue right from the building design phase represents an extraordinary opportunity for implementing a "zero-lift" approach. Since the direct and indirect costs of occupational injuries are very high, investments made at the outset have a good chance of achieving rapid self-financing.

The equipment-purchasing program should therefore be updated when the recommended equipment has not been planned for. The wide range of transfer equipment currently available on the market has become much more effective, thanks to the efforts made by the suppliers who are more attentive to user needs. One particular example is the ceiling lift.

Recent studies have shown that the results of extensive use of ceiling lifts is very significant in terms of reducing the incidence and seriousness of injuries related to patient transfers. These studies also show that it is possible to completely self-finance these installations over a 5-year period exclusively through savings in compensation to occupational accident victims (Engst, Chhokar, Miller, & Yassi, 2004; Villeneuve, 1999; Villeneuve, Goumain, & Elabidi, 1994). Furthermore, a ceiling lift can free up floor space.

BARRIER-FREE STANDARDS

We consulted the principal standards for building accessibility in Canada and the US (AIA, 2001; Corporation Hébergement Québec, 1995; Department of Veterans Affairs, 2004). These standards represent significant social progress in that they allow handicapped people to enjoy a more active life. They prescribe the *minimum conditions* for building access, by requiring a barrier-free route from the parking lot to points of service. An important limitation, however, is that these standards are designed for handicapped people in wheelchairs who have enough arm strength to get around on their own or to transfer independently. Unfortunately, this does not correspond to the profile of most hospital patients, and even less so to long-term care facilities, where the majority of patients need partial or complete assistance with their transfers. The availability of one or more caregivers using specialized equipment is required. To perform transfers without risk of injury to either the patient or the caregiver, an appropriate space must be available. Those standards do not take into account the real work situation of caregivers with dependent patients. However, there is no reason as to why we cannot make recommendations that exceed these minimal standards if needed.

SAFE WORKSPACE

A series of typical patient transfer situations is illustrated. We feel that the recommended workspace in each case is realistic. The proposed room designs were the subject of dynamic simulations for several construction projects and were validated by users after the fact. The drawings are accompanied by examples of the plan. Basic information about doors, corridors, and ramp dimensions are also available.

The criteria selected to determine useful workspace are based on the amount of space required for typical work activities (see Table 12.1) and the dimensions of commonly used equipment (see Table 12.2).

The addition of 300-mm (12") space around the furniture for bariatric patients is a minimum. It is justified by the difference in the width and length of standard equipment versus those for bariatric patients.

Following are drawings and specifications:

TABLE 12.1 Workspace for Typical Working Activities

Type of Task	Workspace
1. One person working (front)	Minimum 810 mm (32"); better 1000 mm (39")
2. One person working (side)	Minimum 610 mm (24"); better 760 mm (30")
3. Pivot 180° standard wheel chair	1500 mm (5")
4. Pivot 180° floor lift	1800 mm (6'); bariatric floor lift 2440 mm (8')
5. Pivot 180° stand lift	1800 mm (6')
6. Pivot 180° geriatric chair	1800 mm (6')
7. Pivot 180° stretcher	2400 mm (8')
8. Circulation space, standard wheelchair	915 mm (36"); better 1000 mm (39")
9. Circulation space, stretcher	915 mm (36"); better 1000 mm (39")
10. Circulation space, bed (standard)	1060 mm (42"); better 1220 mm (48")

N.B. To be safe, add a minimum of 300 mm (12") to the workspace where bariatric patients are moved (see Table 12.2). There are also some obese employees who need more working space.

TABLE 12.2   Equipment—Overall Dimensions

Equipment	Standard		Bariatric		Difference	
	Width	Length	Width	Length	Width	Length
Bed	1000 mm (39")	2260 mm (89")	1000–1370 mm (39"–54")	2220–2444 mm (88"–96")	380 mm (15")	229 mm (9")
Restchair	640 mm (26")	810 mm (32")	810 mm (32")	915 mm (36")	150 mm (6")	100 mm (4")
Stretcher	810 mm (32")	1980 mm (78")	960 mm (38")	2080 mm (82")	150 mm (6")	100 mm (4")
Floor lift	630 mm (25"); 1120 mm (44") base open	1245 mm (49")	630 mm (25"); 1980 mm (78") base open	1245 mm (49"); 1625 mm (64") base open	864 mm (34")	380 mm (15")
Wheelchair	700 mm (28")	1220 mm (48")	850 mm (34")	1320 mm (52")	150 mm (6")	100 mm (4")
Electric wheelchair	820 mm (32")	1060 mm (42")	1000 mm (39")	1120 mm (44")	180 mm (7")	60 mm (2.5")
Commode/showerchair	450 mm (24")	400 mm (24")	760 mm (30")	760 mm (30")	150 mm (6")	150 mm (6")
Transfer bathchair	760 mm (30")	530 mm (21")	915 mm (36")	610 mm (24")	150 mm (6")	40 mm (3")

N.B.

1. Overall dimensions may vary with companies. Values are approximate.
2. Bariatric equipment is about 150 mm (6")–380 mm (15") *wider* and from 40 mm (3") to 229 mm (9") *longer* except for a floor lift. A bariatric floor lift is 864 mm (34") *wider* and 380 mm (15") *longer* and requires 2440 mm (96") free floor space. A ceiling lift is more convenient for bariatric patients.
3. Add a minimum of 300 mm (12") to the workspace where bariatric equipment is used. For a bariatric floor lift add a minimum of 600 mm (24").

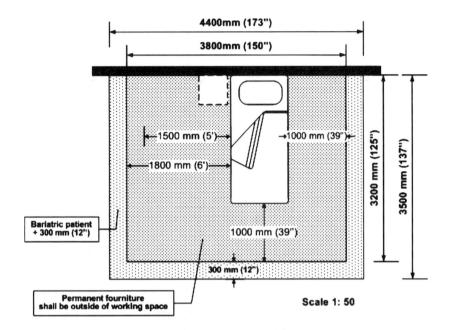

The working space includes at least 810 mm (32') for the care giver and the equipment used to transfert the patient

➢ Transfert bed/wheelchair or bed/stretcher: 1500 mm (5')

➢ Transfert with floor lift or bed/geriatric chair: 1800 mm (6')
   N.B. Ceilling-lift could saves about 300 mm (12") floor space with a transfert to wheelchair and is more efficient than floor lift

➢ Space for care giver and restchair: 1000 mm (39")
   N.B. Transfert bed/restchair should be made on the larger side of the bed and then roll the chair near the windows

➢ Circulation at the foot of the bed: 1000 mm (39")

➢ Bariatric patient: add 300 mm (12") all around the bed, equipments are bigger

➢ Door room width: 1100 mm (43") standard, 1220 mm (48") for Bariatric patient and easier to roll in/out medical equipment

➢ Working space:
   Standard: 12 sqm (127 sqft)
   Bariatric: 15 sqm (158 sqft)
   N.B. Surface may be larger with a wider or longer bed

FIGURE 12.3   Working space—transfer to bed.

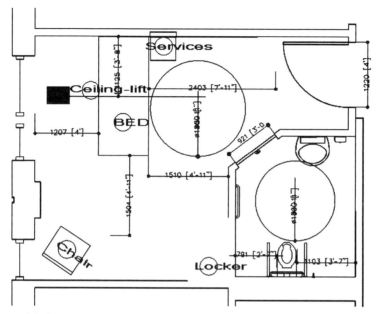

Single bedroom including a wheelchair accessible bathroom.

Room space: net surface, approximately 17 sqm (180 sqft), depending on the configuration of the space

➤ Access to the bed on three sides.

➤ Space around the bed:
- On the side nearest the door (principal workspace): 1800 mm (6') for a transfer involving a floor lift or geriatric chair; 2100 mm available for bariatric patient transfer
- Window side (secondary workspace): 1200 mm (47") working space
- Foot of the bed (traffic area): 1200 mm (47") circulation space

➤ Ceiling lift installed over the bed preferable to a floor lift

➤ Control panel (medical gases, call bell, etc.) on the door side; preferably on the patient's right side because doctors usually examine patients on this side

➤ Room door: minimum width 1220 mm (48"). Should be wide enough to accommodate a bed and equipment into the room; no threshold.

➤ Movable bedside table to facilitate transfers to a stretcher or positioning of the client in the bed.

➤ Cupboard for the client's personal effects; could also hold the TV.

Characteristic of this model of room: The bed faces the door. Advantages: much more free space on the transfer side; better client supervision. Privacy can be provided by angling the door and closing the curtain.

Bathroom space: net surface, approximately 4.5 sqm (48 sqft), depending on the configuration of the space

➤ Door: 915 mm (36") wide.

➤ Toilet out from adjacent walls and equipped with retractable bars attached to the wall for client transfers assisted by one or two caregivers.

➤ 610 mm (24") minimum clearance on each side of the toilet (person standing), 915 mm (width of a standard WC), 1100 mm (length of a standard WC)

➤ Wheelchair-accessible sink.

➤ WC rotation: 1500 mm (5') diameter.

➤ Non-skid, easy-clean floor.

➤ Floor drain in the event of overflow.

➤ No threshold.

FIGURE 12.4 Example of a universal single bedroom layout.

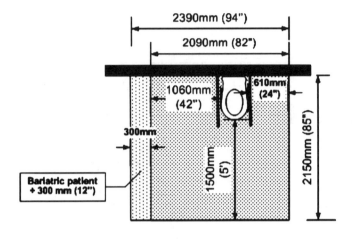

Scale 1: 50

➢ Space for care giver on both sides of toilet to assist the patient: minimum 610 mm (24")

➢ Wall movable handrail on both sides of toilet

➢ Space for a « pivot transfert » at 90o in front of toilet and for a « lateral transfert » on one side : 1060 mm (42")

➢ Space to move equipement in front of toilet: 1500 mm (5')

➢ Bariatric patient: add 300 mm (12") on the side of the transfert

➢ Door width: 810 mm (32") standard, 915 mm (36") and better 1100 (43") for bariatric patient; easier to roll in/out equipment

➢ Sliding door saves space inside the washroom

➢ Working space:
　　Standard: 4.5 sqm (48 sqft)
　　Bariatric: 5 sqm (53 sqft)
　　N.B. Surface may varies with toilet overall dimensions

FIGURE 12.5   Working space—transfer to toilet.

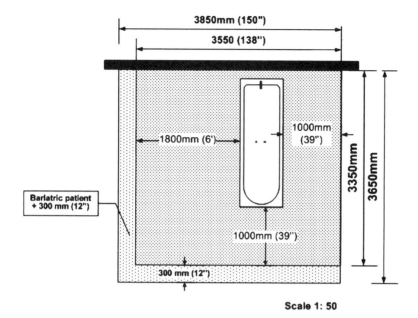

Scale 1: 50

The working space includes at least 810 mm (32') for the care giver and the equipment used to transfert the patient

➢ Transfert with bath chair or stretcher by the side : 1800 mm (6'); add 300 mm (12") for bariatric patient
N.B. Transfert made by the foot of the bath tub: 1800 mm (6'); Ceiling-lift could save about 300 mm (12") floor space

➢ Space for care giver: 1000 mm (39")

➢ Circulation at the foot of the bath tub: 1000 mm (39"); add 300 mm (12") for bariatric patient

➢ Door width: 915 mm (36") standard, 1100 mm (43") for bariatric patient and easier to roll in/out transfert equipment

➢ Working space:
Standard: 12 sqm (127 sqft)
Bariatric: 14 sqm (148 sqft)
N.B. Surface may varies with bath tub overall dimensions

FIGURE 12.6   Working space—transfer to bath tub.

CLINICAL BATHROOM

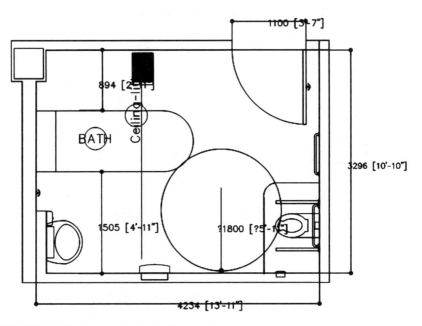

FIGURE 12.7   Example of a bathroom layout.

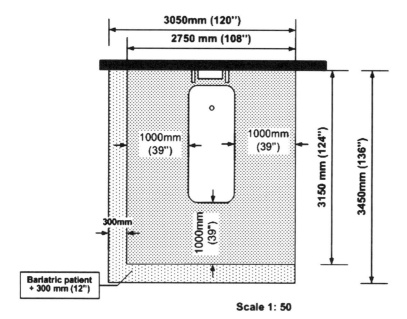

Scale 1: 50

The working space includes at least 810 mm (32') for the care giver and the equipment used to transfert the patient

➤ Space for care giver right/left side and at the foot of the trolley: 1000 mm (39")

➤ Bariatric patient: add 300 mm (12") on transfert side and at the foot of trolley

➤ Door width: 915 mm (36") standard, 1100 mm (43") for bariatric patient and easier to roll in/out equipment

➤ Working space:
   Standard: 9 sqm (95 sqft)
   Bariatric: 11 sqm (116 sqft)
   N.B. Surface may varies with shower trolley overall dimensions

FIGURE 12.8   Working space—transfer with shower trolley.

HANDICAPED SHOWER

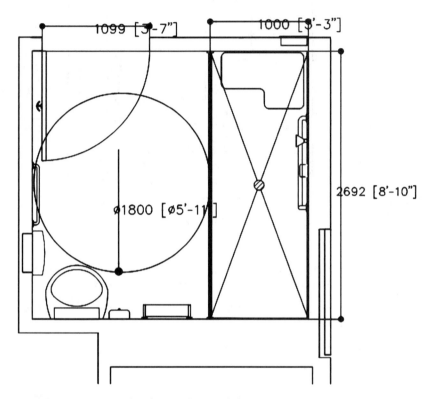

FIGURE 12.9   Example of a handicapped shower.

DOORS

DIMENSIONS

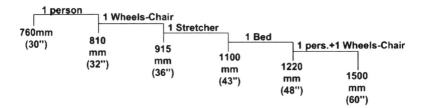

CORRIDORS

DIMENSIONS

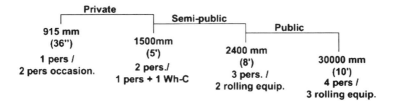

RAMPS

DIMENSIONS (feet)

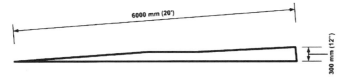

> ➢ **Avoid ramps. If not possible, ramps ratio 1:20**
> ➢ **Ramps ratio 1:12 is too difficult for elderly people**
> ➢ **Provide a midway step rest on the ramps**

FIGURE 12.10   Specifications for doors, corridors, and ramps.

REFERENCES

ASSTSAS (1992). *L'ergonomie appliquée aux services de santé*, Actes du colloque. www.asstsas.qc.ca

Engst, C., Chhokar, R., Miller, A., & Yassi, A. (2004). Preventing back injuries to healthcare workers in British Columbia, Canada and the ceiling lift experience. In W. Charney, & A. Hudson (Eds.), *Back injury among healthcare workers* (Chap. 15, pp. 253–263). New York, NY: Lewis Publishers.

Owen, B. D. (2004). Magnitude of the problem. In W. Charney, & A. Hudson (Eds.), *Back injury among healthcare workers* (Chap. 2, pp. 5–12). New York, NY: Lewis Publishers.

Stubbs, D. A., Buckle P. W., Hudson, M. P., & Rivers, P. M. (1983). Back pain in nursing profession. II. Epidemiology and pilot methodology. *Ergonomics, 26*, 775–765.

St. Vincent, M., Lortie, M., & Tellier, C. (1987). A new approach for the evaluation of training programs in safe lifting. In S. Asfour (Ed.), *Trends in ergonomics/human factors IV* (pp. 847–855). Holland: Elsevier Science Publishers B.V.

Villeneuve, J. (2000). Ergonomic design in health care facilities: a user-focused approach. *Journal of Healthcare Safety, Compliance & Infection Control, 4*(3), 107–144.

Villeneuve, J. (2004). Participatory ergonomic design in health care facilities. In W. Charney, & A. Hudson (Eds.), *Back injury among healthcare workers* (Chap. 11, pp. 161–178). New York, NY: Lewis Publishers.

Villeneuve, J. (1999). The ceiling-lift: An efficient way of preventing injuries among nursing staff. In W. Charney (Ed.), *Handbook of modern hospital safety* (part 3, pp. 736–741). New York, NY: Lewis Publishers.

Villeneuve, J., Goumain, P., & Elabidi, D. (1994). A comparative study of two types of patient-lifting devices for moving patients in long-term care, *Proceedings of the International Ergonomics Association (IEA) Conference*, Toronto, Canada.

Zimring, C. (1997). Site visits. In S. O. Marberry (Ed.), *Healthcare design* (pp. 3–25). Indianapolis, IN: John Wiley & Sons.

STANDARDS AND GUIDELINES

AIA (The American Institute of Architects), Guidelines for Design and Construction of Hospital and Health Care Facilities, 2001. In revision cycle. www.aia.org

CAN/CSA-B651-95, Barrier-Free Design, Canadian Standards Association, 1995. www.csa.ca

Corporation Hébergement Québec, Cadre de référence normatif, 2004. www.chq.gouv.qc.ca

Department of Veterans Affairs, Barrier Free Design Guide, PG-18-13, Office of Facilities Management, October 2004. www.index.va.gov

Uniform Federal Accessibility Standards (UFAS), ADA Accessibility Guidelines for buildings and Facilities (ADAAG). www.accessboard.gov

CHAPTER THIRTEEN

Ergonomic Workplace Assessments of Patient Handling Environments

Guy Fragala and Audrey L. Nelson

One of the first steps in preventing occupational injuries is to study the workplace for the presence of risk factors. Once a job-related risk factor is identified in the workplace, the hazard should be analyzed and a method to improve the job needs to be developed. Through the principles of ergonomics, jobs can be redesigned and improved to be within reasonable limits of human capabilities. The basic principles of ergonomics offer the best hope in improving the problems associated with occupational musculoskeletal disorders associated with patient handling tasks. The purpose of this chapter is to present a protocol for conducting an ergonomic assessment of patient care environments.

ERGONOMIC SYSTEMS APPROACH

An ergonomic systems approach is used to analyze job tasks and identify prominent risk factors with the purpose of changing unacceptable job

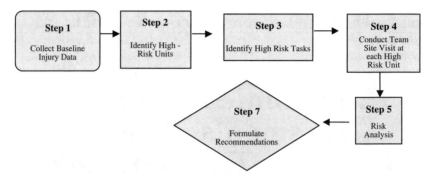

FIGURE 13.1   Overview of ergonomic workplace assessment protocol for patient care environments.

demands. Specifically, ergonomic approaches are used to:

- Design jobs and job tasks to fit people rather than expecting people to adapt to poor work designs.
- Achieve a proper match between the worker and their job by understanding and incorporating the limits of people.
- Take into account that problems will occur when job demands exceed the limits of care providers.

A summary of the ergonomic environment assessment protocol for patient care units can be found in Figure 13.1. Each step will be described.

Step 1—Collect Baseline Injury Data

Injury data should focus on injuries related to patient handling and movement. Each clinical unit should gather and record their individual information. Data should minimally capture a description of the incident including the patient care activity performed at the time of the injury, time of the incident, unit/location where incident occurred, body parts affected, days of work lost, and modified duty days.

Step 2—Identify High-Risk Units

Using baseline data on the incidence and severity of injuries identify the high-risk units at the facility. Eventually, every patient care area will be included in the ergonomic assessment process, but prioritization is important to effectively allocate available resources. High-risk units will normally have the highest incidence of patient handling injuries, the most workdays lost, and the highest concentration of staff on modified duty.

Step 3—Identify High-Risk Tasks

Next, it is important to identify and assess staff perceptions of high-risk tasks. The highest risk tasks are likely to vary between patient care units, depending on patient characteristics, availability of equipment, physical layout, and work organization. For example, some studies have indicated that bathing tasks, toileting tasks and transfers from beds to chairs are high-stress tasks for patient handlers. Other units may prioritize lateral transfers from bed to stretcher, or turning patients from side to side in bed.

Through job observation, questionnaires to employees or brainstorming sessions with patient handlers, individual sites should determine what are the high-risk activities within their organization. Figure 13.2 is a tool that can be used with nursing staff to identify and prioritize high-risk tasks.

It is important to include as many direct patient care providers as possible in delineating high-risk tasks. Keep in mind that there are likely to be variations by unit as well as by shift.

Step 4—Conduct Team Site Visit for Ergonomic Assessment

This site evaluation serves to recognize many direct and indirect factors that may contribute to risk potential and, with staff input, to identify potential solutions that will serve to minimize risk of injury to the caregivers and patients.

Generally the site visit team will evaluate equipment availability and use, space issues, storage availability, and maintenance/repair issues. Other factors such as patient population and staffing information are needed to determine unit characteristics that will influence intervention needs.

Plan a brief meeting with the manager on the unit. During this meeting, staffing levels, scheduling practices, and patient assignments are revisited in which we learn about:

1. Ceiling and typical patient census
2. Staffing levels by shift
3. Unique shift patterns
4. Typical number of staff on modified or light duty assignment
5. Staff turnover
6. Peak workload periods
7. Workload distribution using special teams such as shower or lift teams

Directions: Assign a rank (from 1 to 10) to the tasks you consider to be the highest risk tasks contributing to musculoskeletal injuries for persons providing direct patient care. A "1" should represent the highest risk, "2" for the second highest, etc. For each task, consider the frequency of the task (high, moderate, low) and musculoskeletal stress (high, moderate, low) of each task when assigning a rank. Delete tasks not typically performed on your unit. You can have each nursing staff member complete the form and summarize the data, or you can have staff work together by shift to develop the rank by consensus.

Frequency of Task	Stress of Task	Rank	Patient Handling Tasks
H = High	H = High	1 = High-Risk	
M = Moderate	M = Moderate		
L = Low	L = Low	10 = Low Risk	
			Transferring patient from bathtub-to-chair.
			Transferring patient from wheelchair or shower/commode chair to bed.
			Transferring patient from wheelchair-to-toilet.
			Transferring a patient from bed-to-stretcher.
			Lifting a patient up from the floor.
			Weighing a patient.
			Bathing a patient in bed.
			Bathing a patient in a shower chair.
			Bathing a patient on a shower trolley or stretcher.
			Undressing/dressing a patient.
			Applying anti-embolism stockings.
			Lifting patient to the head of the bed.
			Repositioning patient in bed from side-to-side.
			Repositioning patient in geriatric chair or wheelchair.
			Making an occupied bed.
			Feeding bed-ridden patient.
			Changing absorbent pad.
			Transporting patient off unit.
			Other Task:

Adapted from Owen, B.D. & Garg, A. (1991). *AAOHN Journal, 39,* **(1).**

FIGURE 13.2   Tool for prioritizing high-risk patient handling tasks.

Once you have the group of staff convened, solicit staff input into risks related to patient care activities. Samples of general questions are outlined below.

- What conditions or situations put you at risk to back strain and injuries?
- Which lifts or transfers are the most difficult and present the highest risk?
- What are the factors that make a lift or transfer a high-risk activity?
- What types of patient conditions contribute to high-risk situations?
- What do you think can be done to reduce or minimize a high-risk situation?
- How can we more effectively use lifting aid devices?
- What are the important features to look for in a lifting aid device?

With a more complete understanding of operational issues specific to the unit, the ergonomics team requests a guided tour of the unit. During this tour, the team pays particular attention to:

- The availability, size, and configuration of storage space
- Showering/bathing processes and equipment
- Toileting processes and equipment
- Patient room sizes and configurations
- Provision and condition of equipment for patient transfer, including mechanical lifts, stand assist lifts, lateral transfer aids, etc.

Information derived from the site visits is compiled, by unit, into a summary data sheet (Figure 13.3). On this data sheet, the patient population and unit type are described, along with miscellaneous pertinent information, such as future plans of the unit. Availability and condition of equipment on-hand are noted. Problems identified by the ergonomics team are recorded in detail, allowing for the development and recording of proposed solutions.

Step 5—Risk Analysis

Risk analysis involves careful review of the baseline injury data, identification of high-risk tasks, and observational data from the site visit. In this step, a determination is made as to what changes are required for improvement.

Risk factors specific to the healthcare industry might include:

- Reaching and lifting with loads far from the body
- Lifting heavy loads
- Twisting while lifting

Unit: _____

Patient Description	Unit Description	Misc. Info.	Equipment	Problems Identified	Solutions
Sample:					
Spinal Cord Injury – includes new injuries and 4-6 ventilator dependent patients. 60% of patients are totally dependent.	This 34-bed SCI unit has two wings, 7 private rooms, 3 semi-private and 5 three-bed rooms. Showers are communal (2 areas), as are bathrooms.	Unit will be moving in 8 months.	3 ARJO Maxilifts. TotalLift II. Not Used: Mobilizer, Surfboard.	Most of injuries are from repositioning patient in bed. Lateral transfers are also problematic, and there is no equipment staff has found useful. No preventative maintenance program for equipment. One additional lift needed for peak periods on each shift; batteries on existing lifts are old, and not all lifts have scales. New batteries, two XXL slings, and one scale for ARJO Lift.	Pneu-Care mattresses for 10 beds – or – ceiling lift with clamps on sheets to pull patient up in bed – or – parachute material for sheets. Get estimate of current mattress expenditures, and get turn-assist or rotational therapy added on. Explore best surface for pulling up in bed. Two Gait belts with handles. One powered, lateral-assist device. Explore value of friction reducing devices. Additional Maxi Lift with scale. Preventative maintenance program needed.

FIGURE 13.3   Sample summary data from site visit.

- Unexpected changes in load demand during the lift
- Reaching low or high to begin a lift
- Moving/carrying a load a significant distance

Environmental hazards are also identified, such as cluttered patient care areas, confined space in bathrooms, or broken equipment.

To achieve improvement related to reducing musculoskeletal disorders among healthcare workers involved in direct patient care, difficult and demanding jobs must be redesigned applying the principles and concepts of ergonomics. High-risk jobs must be changed and modified and a strategy for redesigning jobs as follows is suggested:

1. Can the need to do the high-risk activity be eliminated, such as by eliminating a bed-to-chair transfer using a bed which converts into a chair configuration?
2. Can the high-risk activity be redesigned using devices such as mechanical lifts?
3. Can the high-risk activity be improved through risk reduction using some type of lifting aid device, such as a gait belt with handles or friction-reducing sheet?

In order to effectively integrate new and improved job design into the process of delivering care within healthcare facilities, a basic structure or process can contribute to the level of improvement achieved. A simple structure for the ergonomic management process is as follows:

1. Identify jobs and job tasks, which stress body parts beyond limits
2. Identify and develop solutions to change these task demands
3. Use a well-thought-out process to implement these changes into the workplace
4. In addition to reviewing job design, also review the design of the physical work environment to remove barriers, minimize travel, and consider spatial relations

Step 6—Formulate Recommendations

Recommendations should be achievable and simple. When developing recommendations it is necessary to factor in constraints such as fiscal resources, administrative support, and environment. Generally solutions fall into two categories: engineering controls and administrative controls. Each will be briefly described.

Engineering Design Solutions.   These solutions usually involve a physical change in the way a job task is conducted or physical modification to the workplace. The changes can be observed as caregivers conduct the job task in a new way. Examples might include the introduction of lateral transfer aids, mechanical-lifting aids, height-adjustable beds to match with stretcher heights, or the use of wheelchairs that can be converted into stretchers.

These aids are usually more permanent solutions to problems. They may have a higher initial cost but may have a lower cost over the long term as a result of cost reductions realized from the implementation of the changes.

Through engineering controls, changes are made in job design to minimize or eliminate risk factors. Consider some high-risk patient handling activities with the idea of changing the high-risk components of the job. Tasks involving a bed-to-chair or chair-to-bed transfer can be very difficult. First, consider moving someone out of a bed and into a chair. The difficulty of the task will vary relative to the dependency level of the person to be moved. Considering a totally dependent person, staff members must reach across an obstacle (the bed) to access the person they need to assist. This involves reaching, and it is usually not possible to position oneself with bent knees since the caregiver is usually leaning up against a bed. The patient needs to be physically lifted, and considering weight, the loads involved in the lift are unacceptable. Movement into a chair involves moving the person to a different height level, and there is usually some carrying involved. The unacceptable risk factors of this job task involve reaching, lifting a heavy load, sub optimal lifting postures, and carrying a load a significant distance. In order to redesign this task effectively, the optimum solution would be to eliminate these high-risk activities. Where task elimination is not an option, lifting aid devices can be applicable to this situation. Lifting aid devices include full-body slings, which are very useful for the totally dependent patient. In addition, the bed-to-chair transfer can be converted into a bed-to-stretcher transfer. Through the use of convertible wheelchairs that bend back and convert into stretchers and with height adjustment capabilities, a slide transfer rather than a lift may result.

If the patient is not totally dependent, a transfer such as bed to chair may be done by first getting the patient to a sitting posture. Again the amount of assistance required will depend upon the patient's status. Once to a sitting posture, a stand and pivot transfer can be conducted. Some healthcare workers are highly skilled in this transfer technique and have done it many times without suffering from any occupational injuries. However, loads involved are heavy and if the patient does something unexpectedly, such as collapses from a weakness in the legs, the healthcare worker must react and often these unexpected occurrences can result in occupational injuries. Again through application of some lifting aid devices, the risk associated with this type of transfer can be minimized. A device that could be considered in this situation would be a standing and repositioning lift, which is a lifting device with a simpler sling for patients with weight-bearing capabilities.

Administrative Solutions. These usually involve the caregivers only in the way the work is done and do not involve a physical change to the workplace. Changes are apparent by watching how the work is conducted or how caregivers perform their jobs. Examples might include changes in scheduling, minimizing the amount of times a patient or resident must be transferred, job rotation where more people are involved in the process of transfers, or the introduction of lifting teams.

These recommendations are usually relatively fast and easy to implement and may have a low initial cost. However, implementation requires continual enforcement and reenforcement and, although short-term successes may be realized, it is difficult to achieve long-term change and improvement.

Administrative controls may be applied to patient handling tasks. For example, the number of patient transfers may be reduced by effectively scheduling procedures that patients may require over the day. Rather than transferring patients from a bed to a wheelchair or transport device for a particular procedure or diagnostic test and then bringing them back to their room, putting them back to bed, and redoing the transfer for a number of other procedures during the day, scheduling could be planned better. Scheduling might be done so that the patients will be transferred out of bed, brought from place to place for various necessary procedures, and then returned to their room.

Here is an example of how administrative controls can be used, involving rescheduling to minimize a high concentration of lifting activities for direct patient care staff. It takes place at a state department for the developmentally disabled involving facilities for housing highly dependent patients who are in need of much assistance to be moved. One of the most demanding times for patient transfers involved the part of the day when staff members were preparing patients to be picked up in buses and transported to their daily activities. Because of the way activities were scheduled and how the buses ran, staff members were rushing and highly stressed to prepare patients for transport in a short time period. Lifting aid equipment was considered and did improve the situation; however, the short window of time to get patients out of bed and prepared for transport was creating the problem. This was not an issue that staff caring for the patients could solve themselves. It involved many people throughout the entire facility, including those responsible for scheduling patient activity programs and meals, as well as the organization that had been contracted to provide transport services. Other than the direct patient care staff, the other groups were unaware of the problems encountered with the short time window provided to prepare patients for transport. After an initial meeting was held with these other operational groups at the facility, they understood the problem and were more than willing to consider options to improve the situation. Scheduled activities were adjusted and methods of transport pickups were also changed. This resulted in distributing the number of required transfers over a larger period of the workday and allowed for better use of lifting aid equipment. The implementation of this administrative control required some careful planning and presentation of the problem as well as cooperation from a wide segment of many operational groups within the facility. The end results were positive to all involved including the patients, who received better care. This was due to the fact that direct patient care staff had more time in preparation for the transport process and they could give more individual attention to patients.

OTHER KEY FACTORS TO CONSIDER

Assessment should include direct patient care providers' participation in evaluating risks in nursing work environments. Key roles for direct care providers include:

- Identification of the most stressful job tasks
- Evaluation of suggested solutions to problems including patient transferring procedures and devices
- Selection of the most effective procedures and devices, and participation in implementation of the program
- Input on injury investigation making employees equal partners where they will take ownership of the program as much as possible

Assessment should include managers' participation in evaluating risks in nursing work environments. Key roles for managers include:

- Encourage worker participation so that they will feel confident and perform well
- Emphasize positive reinforcement
- Appreciate and respect employees for achieving small goals
- Seek workers input prior to any decision making
- Good communication where information and feedback are provided in a timely manner
- Address workers' problems and concerns

Table 13.1 depicts a series of case studies where patient care ergonomic assessment protocols were successfully implemented.

TABLE 13.1 Case Studies of Successful Patient Care Ergonomic Assessments

Site	Assessment approach	Problems identified	Solution	Results
BJC Health System Nursing Homes [460 direct patient care staff at 6 sites] (Collins, Wolf, & Hsiao, 2002)	• Examined injury data; all nursing home units were considered to be high risk • Identified high-risk tasks on each unit	Identified high-risk activities included: transfers in and out of bed; in and out of bath tubs, showers and whirlpools; on and off toilets; repositioning in bed; and lifting a resident who has collapsed from the floor	• A zero-lift policy that uses state-of-the-art equipment to assist with patient transfers • Training in the use of patient transferring equipment • A medical management program for safely returning injured workers to patient care	Over a 3-year period: • Lifting-related injuries decreased by 51.8% • Injury incidence rate decreased by 49.7% • Injury costs decreased by 61.2%
Seven nursing homes located in four (4) different states, and one hospital in Canada [1446 employees] (Garg, 1999)	• Examined injury statistics including number of injuries, lost workdays and workers' compensation cost • Active caregiver and manager participation in process	Manual lifting and transferring of patients were the most hazardous tasks in their facilities. The targeted tasks included lifting and transferring patients from bed to wheelchair, wheelchair to bed, bed or wheelchair to toilet, toilet to bed for wheelchair, lifting patients off the floor, bed or wheelchair to bathtub, shower chair or gurney and	• Zero-lift programs were implemented by replacing manual lifting and transferring of patients with modern, battery operated portable lifts, and other patient transfer assist devices • Adequate staffing was provided • Hired an ergonomics coordinator	• The number of injuries decreased by 62% • Lost workdays decreased by 86% • Restricted workdays decreased by 64% • Worker's compensation costs decreased by 84% • Intangible benefits included improvements in patients comfort and safety during transfers and patient care *(Continued)*

TABLE 13.1 (Continued)

Site	Assessment approach	Problems identified	Solution	Results
Masonic home and hospital, Wallingford, Connecticut [1200 employees] (Fragala, 1995a)	• The Assistant Director of Human Resources championed the assessment and an initiation team was developed, including front line care providers • Workers' Compensation Trust provided strong support in analyzing injury data • Through facility tours and brainstorming sessions, high-risk areas were identified	back, weighing patients, and bathing. In addition, some nursing homes also targeted repositioning in bed and wheelchair • The team found no correlation between staffing patterns or long shifts to the rate of injuries • Manual patient lifting was the primary risk identified • While equipment was available, staff were not using it	• Training, monitoring, feedback to employees • Injury investigation and medical management • Purchased lifting aid devices • The Initiation Team now became an Implementation Team or a Continuous Quality Improvement Team, and they appointed contact people on each unit who were responsible for making sure staff felt comfortable using the new equipment • Continuous Quality Improvement Team members also toured the facility and spoke at staff meetings, particularly those team members who were	• Annual lost workdays decreased by 92.1% • Incurred annual workers' compensation costs decreased by 77.2%

Lawrence and
Memorial Hospital,
New London,
Connecticut
[1400 employees]
(Fragala &
Santamaria, 1997)

Nurse Managers
were asked to hold
brainstorming
sessions with staff
members to gather
information and
a back injury
questionnaire was
sent out to all
nursing staff. From
the data gathered,
four main reasons
were identified as
perceived to be
important when
considering causes,
which contribute
to back injuries
due to lifting
patients

- Causes of job-related
  patient handling injuries
  were identified as:
- Low staffing levels
- No time to wait for help,
  that is, rushing to the next
  patient, late lunch, or
  getting near the end of a
  work shift
- Current lifting aid equipment available to assist in
  patient lifts was difficult to
  use and not readily available
- The nature of the work
  itself was difficult even
  when adequate staff are
  available such as three or
  four nurses to assist in a
  lifting task; someone was
  still at risk for injury
- The Orthopedic Unit was
  found to have the highest

Certified Nursing
Assistants themselves
- Introduced an ergo-
  nomic management
  program

Once problems were
identified and pri-
orities set as to
which units or floors
needed attention,
work began on re-
designing high-risk
activities. Through a
categorization of the
patient population
in the Orthopedic
Unit and the Medical
Surgical Unit, it was
determined that if
two types of patient
lifting aid devices
were obtained, many
of the unacceptable
job tasks could be
changed. The devices
identified were a
standing and reposi-
tioning lifting aid

- Number of injuries
  decreased by 75.0%
- Number of lost
  workdays decreased by
  100%
- Number of restricted
  days decreased by
  98.4%
- Indemnity costs
  decreased by 99.7%
- Replacement costs
  decreased by 100%

(Continued)

TABLE 13.1 *(Continued)*

Site	Assessment approach	Problems identified	Solution	Results
		number of lost workdays and restricted workdays and Medical Surgical was found to have the highest number of back injuries due to patient lifting. In the Orthopedic Unit, 50% of the back injuries were due to boosting patients ups in bed and 50% due to chair-to-bed transfers • In the Medical Surgical Unit, chair-to-bed transfer was identified as a high-risk activity with 50% of injuries attributable to this activity	with a commode attachment and a full-body sling lift with a bed scale attachment. Although funds had not been budgeted for expenditures such as patient lifting aid equipment, support from senior management had been established and when the request for funds to purchase these engineering controls was made, the request was approved and funds were provided through a contingency fund to purchase needed patient lifting aid devices	

REFERENCES

Collins, J. W., Wolf, L., & Hsiao, H. (2002). Intervention Program for Transferring Residents in Nursing Homes. Centers for Disease Control and Prevention, National Institute for Occupational Safety and Health, BJC Health System. Presented at Safe Patient Handling and Movement Conference, Tampa, FL.

Fragala, G. (1995a). Ergonomics: the essential element for effective back injury prevention for healthcare workers. *American Society of Safety Engineers, March*, 23–25.

Fragala, G., & Santamaria, D. (1997). Heavy duties? *Health Facilities Management, May*, 22–27.

Garg, A. (1999). Long-Term Effectiveness of "Zero-Lift Program" in Seven Nursing Homes and One Hospital. U.S. Department of Health & Human Services, Center for Disease Control and Prevention. August 16; Contract No. U60/CCU512089-02.

Owen, B. D., Garg, A. (1991). Reducing risk for back pain in nursing personnel. *AAOHN Journal, 39*(1), 24–33.

PART IV

Future Directions

CHAPTER FOURTEEN

Being a Change Agent and Advocate for Safe Patient Handling

Laureen G. Doloresco

Staff nurses can be powerful catalysts for improving safe patient handling in their practice settings. Frontline nurses are ideally positioned to identify hazardous patient handling tasks, redesign work processes, and make recommendations for patient care equipment. By applying concepts from planned change theory, nurses can compel their organization to take action to create safer patient care environments.

LEWIN'S THEORY OF PLANNED CHANGE

Successful change agents use a systematic planning process to gain support for new ideas, procedures, and technology. Kurt Lewin's theory of planned change (1947) provides a practical model that can easily be applied by nurses to effect improvements in patient handling. Change is described as a dynamic process resulting from competing forces in the environment. Driving forces are factors that propel change. Restraining forces are factors that act as barriers to change and maintain the status quo. Together,

"The views expressed in this article are those of the author and do not necessarily represent the view of the Department of Veterans Affairs. No claim made to U.S. government material. Contact Author: Laureen.Doloresco@med.va.gov."

driving and restraining forces interact within a force field to create a state of equilibrium. For change to occur, the force field must be altered by either reducing restraining forces or increasing driving forces.

An analysis of driving and restraining forces is essential before nurses can initiate a change to improve safe patient handling practices. For example, restraining forces related to installation of ceiling-mounted lifts on a spinal cord injury rehabilitation unit may include beliefs by clinical staff that the technology is incongruent with the goal of promoting the patient's maximal independence. Another restraining force may be the view by hospital administrators that a ceiling lift system is too costly. Nurses can lessen these restraining forces by citing evidence of the successful use of ceiling lifts in other facilities and describing cost savings associated with fewer work-related injuries. Driving forces that support implementation of ceiling-mounted lifts may include a high incidence of nursing injuries, or an increase in patient skin abrasions resulting from manual patient handling tasks. These data provide powerful justification for ceiling lifts.

Lewin's model of planned change identifies three phases: (1) unfreezing an existing situation from a state of equilibrium where driving and restraining forces are in balance; (2) moving to a new level; and (3) refreezing at the new level. Before a change can be made, it is necessary to "unfreeze" the current situation. This involves motivating a target audience to adopt new attitudes, beliefs, or behaviors. During this phase, there is an increasing awareness of a problem and need for a change. The task of a change agent is to help guide this process through communication with stakeholders who will be affected by the change.

Stakeholders include patients, staff, and key leaders who want to know, "What's in it for me?" Enlisting their active participation is critical to minimize resistance and gain maximum "buy in" for the change. The most important element of planned change is the active involvement of affected parties throughout the entire process. The need for a change must be clearly communicated and accepted by those affected by it. Once the target audience is convinced of the need for change, movement to a new level is possible. Refreezing, the final phase in Lewin's model, requires the change agent's continued involvement to ensure that the intervention is implemented according to plans and new behaviors replace those that existed before the change.

SOCIAL MARKETING

Nurses must apply persuasive marketing strategies to implement safe patient handling initiatives. Development of "no-lift" policies, introduction of costly transfer equipment, and implementation of a back injury resource nurse program are ideas that must be "sold" to a target audience. Social marketing is a process designed to sell ideas to influence a target audience to change behavior (Kotler, Roberto, & Lee, 2002). Use of concepts from social marketing will assist nurses in effecting the behavioral changes that are needed to support ergonomic interventions.

The consumer's perception is the focal point of social marketing. Nurses can gain the consumer's perspective by finding out what patients and staff believe, want, and need to make patient handling and movement safe. To successfully promote projects designed to improve safe patient handling, consideration of the organization's perspective is also important. The organization's perspective is primarily focused on costs and other resource requirements (e.g., product, promotional activities, and participation required).

For example, to gain managerial support for a product evaluation of several types of mechanical lifts, it is important to present a brief overview of the project to principal leaders. This summary should include expected outcomes of the project, staff resources (e.g., evaluation team) needed to support the project, any modifications in the physical environment that will be required, and a detailed description of the mechanical lifts to be evaluated. Sensitivity and consideration of patient and staff needs is the key to securing their involvement in an equipment evaluation. Only patients who are medically stable should be invited to participate in the assessment of different lifts. Additionally, the evaluation should be scheduled during a time frame when nurse staffing is adequate, to provide sufficient time for the staff to provide critical feedback about the various lifting devices.

Marketing approaches are most likely to succeed when consumer and organizational perspectives are aligned as closely as possible. Assessing the readiness of patients, staff, and the organizational climate will enhance the nurse's ability to plan safe patient handling interventions. A unit culture that welcomes new ideas and technology facilitates change and innovation.

Acquiring consumer and organizational support for an ergonomics program requires clear communication of the benefits of safe patient handling, realistic goals and objectives, and outcome measures. Media events and other promotional activities are excellent ways to publicize an injury prevention campaign or patient safety intervention project. A written timeline will clarify goals, objectives, resources, and milestones for gauging the success of the program. Periodic review and revision of the timeline with consumers and key leaders encourages broad support for the program. A detailed evaluation plan keeps the focus on expected outcomes from safe patient handling interventions.

Two critical aspects of the planned change process are (1) determining if the change produced the intended results and (2) communicating outcomes.

STRATEGIES TO PROMOTE SAFE
PATIENT HANDLING

The most effective nurse change agents cultivate collaborative relationships across the organization. There are abundant opportunities for staff nurses to become involved in unit-based and hospital-wide patient safety activities. The following are proactive approaches staff nurses can adopt to increase their visibility as advocates for safe patient handling:

- Present patient handling issues and recommendations to management
- Create a unit-based ergonomics committee
- Serve as a unit resource and peer safety leaders (Matz, in press [a])
- Organize a safe patient handling equipment exhibition
- Volunteer to serve on safety committees and workgroups
- Become active in a professional nursing organization to advocate for an ergonomics approach to patient care
- Facilitate "After-Action Reviews" (AAR) of staff injuries (Matz, in press [b])
- Develop a unit-based Patient Safety Recognition Program

Each of these strategies is discussed below:

Present Patient Handling Issues and
Recommendations to Management

A succinct, one-page memorandum with key points in bulleted format is a convincing way to present specific safety issues and recommendations to nursing and hospital management. This helps to clarify problems, propose solutions, and trigger corrective actions. Documentation of issues is most effective when it includes relevant data (e.g., injury rates) and facts from evidence-based literature and supporting organizations (e.g., American Nurses Association's *Handle with Care* campaign, 2003; de Castro, 2004). Scheduling a follow-up meeting with the Nurse Executive to discuss key points in the memorandum will underscore the importance of staff nurse concerns and facilitate resolution of issues related to safe patient handling.

Create a Unit-Based Ergonomics Committee

Enlisting nursing and interdisciplinary colleagues as members of an ergonomics committee will profile workplace safety in a highly visible manner. Identification of high-risk patient handling tasks and ergonomics solutions is a primary purpose of the committee. To ensure broad representation and diverse perspectives, invite labor partners, managers, and staff as committee members. Physical therapists and other rehabilitation staff are indispensable participants, given their ability to provide a constructive analysis of patient handling tasks and equipment.

Involve nurse co-workers and patients in selecting equipment. Develop educational awareness programs targeting direct care staff, managers, and patients when new equipment is placed in service.

Establish a communication system where staff at all levels can report concerns about patient handling activities, refer recommendations to the committee, and receive timely responses. Other committee responsibilities may include coordination of patient equipment trials and demonstrations, analysis of patient handling injuries, development of educational programs for staff and patients, and creation of ergonomic guidelines based on the unit's patient population.

Serve as a Unit Resource and Peer Safety Leader

Being champions for safe patient handling requires staff nurses to be knowledgeable of current developments in this area and competent in operating lifting and transfer devices. Enthusiastic, well-respected staff nurses are highly effective as unit-based peer leaders in safe patient handling. Their role includes serving as coach and resource on the unit, identifying workplace hazards, and assisting in implementation of interventions in safe patient handling.

Initiate a journal club to infuse new concepts in patient handling on the unit, involving co-workers in the review and discussion of current articles and videos. Engage co-workers in developing patient/family educational tools to describe the benefits of assistive devices and technology and how they contribute to the patient's safety, dignity, and comfort.

Another key responsibility of the unit's safe patient handling resource nurse is to provide hands-on demonstration of equipment for nurses in orientation and annual competency training for experienced staff. Develop an annual competency checklist that requires return demonstrations of equipment use and safe patient handling procedures to reinforce a culture of safety.

Organize an Equipment Exhibition

A demonstration fair with multiple vendors of patient handling equipment provides staff and patients with an opportunity to review the latest products in the marketplace and compare features of various lifting and transfer equipment. Collaborate with managers, engineering, and local contracting representatives to plan a successful equipment exhibition. Prepare a structured evaluation form that nurses and patients can use to provide feedback about each product. At a later date, the equipment with the highest approval ratings can be assessed further on the patient care unit.

Establishing contacts with key vendors provides nurses with the opportunity to discuss equipment design needs and specific features that require modification. Vendors are often willing to provide equipment for trial evaluations on inpatient units. Participate in product evaluations and equipment trials to acquire the knowledge and power to make cogent recommendations for equipment purchases.

Volunteer to Serve on the Safety Committees and Workgroups

Based on their direct link to patients, nurses are viewed as functioning on the "sharp end" of patient care (Institute of Medicine, 2004). The vigilance and insight of staff nurses make them credible members of interdisciplinary safety committees and workgroups tasked with identification and resolution of specific patient safety issues. Direct care nurses are attuned to inherent risks in patient care tasks and flaws in the physical environment, work processes, or equipment design.

Participation on safety committees, root cause analysis teams, and other task forces gives nurses a greater awareness of patient safety issues across the organization, and an opportunity to share ideas with other disciplines, and also promotes interdisciplinary collaborative problem solving to address patient safety issues. A mixture of clinical and administrative staff from a variety of departments, such as nursing, supply, infection control, and engineering, offers the breadth of expertise that is needed to solve workspace design issues and processes that compromise patient and staff safety.

Become Active in a Professional Nursing Organization to Advocate for an Ergonomics Approach to Patient Care

Professional involvement in local chapters of nursing organizations (e.g., American Nurses Association (ANA), Gerontological Nurses Association) provides nurses with an extensive forum for discussing safe patient handling, advocating for legislation, and joining peers to improve nursing practice environments. Submit a poster or paper for presentation at a professional educational conference to share unit-based projects related to patient handling. Examples of topics for presentation include a comparison of lifting devices, initiation of a turning team, or implementation of a unit-based recognition program for safety improvements. Develop a manuscript for publication in a professional nursing journal to communicate these and other workplace interventions.

Take advantage of the specialty organization's e-mail discussion group to network with nursing peers across the country to discuss specific patient handling issues, inquire about types of equipment for specific tasks, and import policies and procedures. To provide factual data and strengthen the case for acquiring new equipment in the workplace to prevent injuries, refer to position statements from nursing organizations, such as ANA's Elimination of Manual Patient Handling to Prevent Work-Related Musculoskeletal Disorders (June, 2003).

Facilitate AARs of Staff Injuries or Near Misses

An AAR is an approach borrowed from the business world and is used to transfer lessons learned from performance of a task in one setting to another setting (Dixon, 2000). When a nurse sustains an on-the-job injury or comes very close to sustaining one, an AAR allows the entire nursing team to apply lessons learned from the incident so that they can avoid injury when they perform the same task in the future.

A well-respected staff nurse with excellent communication skills is ideally suited to facilitate an AAR. Supervisors are not involved in the AAR process, to keep it as informal as possible and encourage a free flow of information among the staff. In contrast with formal injury reporting requirements, AARs are not documented. The goal is to have the work team recognize that mistakes are inevitable occurrences in the workplace that provide a learning opportunity. A non-punitive, blameless attitude to work-related injuries is essential to make an injured co-worker feel comfortable enough to share information regarding the circumstances surrounding the injury.

To maximize the group process, all nursing team members on duty should participate in the AAR. Structure the AAR as a brief, focused brainstorming session in the break room to allow staff to explore factors that led to the injury or "near miss." The AAR also provides staff with an opportunity to show their concern for the injured co-worker. AARs can be held immediately after the incident or scheduled at a later time. High-risk units may prefer to schedule AARs on a routine basis, (e.g., every Tuesday at 11:00 a.m.), to keep injury prevention as a top priority.

The role of the staff nurse facilitator is to guide the discussion by asking team members a series of questions:

1. What factors contributed to this injury that everyone can learn from?
2. What should have happened instead?
3. What accounted for the difference?
4. What actions can be taken to help prevent this from happening again?
5. What do we need to do to follow up on each of these actions, and who will take responsibility for the follow-up?

The facilitator may need to help the team identify problems that are beyond their control and require administrative assistance from the nurse manager. The AAR is a constructive tactic that emphasizes injuries are systemic problems, not individual problems.

A unit's safety performance can always be improved. Units with a strong culture of patient safety view errors as learning opportunities. Encourage co-workers to also use formal procedures to report back strains or other injuries related to patient handling to identify and correct actual and potential hazards that are associated with high-risk patient care activities.

Develop a Unit-Based Patient Safety Recognition Program

Recognizing and rewarding nurses who are involved in safety improvements sends the message that safe patient handling is highly valued on the unit. Collaborate with co-workers and the nurse manager to develop a Patient Safety Recognition Program, establishing a formal process for publicizing staff contributions to patient safety. It is important to recognize and reward individuals and groups who make improvements in work processes as well as those who participate in special projects that result in safety improvements. Examples of staff contributions to patient safety that merit recognition include:

- Organizing patient lifting/transfer equipment and accessories (e.g., slings) in a standard location
- Standardizing patient care assignments so that a nurse does not have more than two successive days of working with a "heavy care," totally dependent patient
- Developing a patient/family educational brochure on the benefits of mechanical aids and equipment for safe patient handling

- Initiating safety rounds to identify environmental hazards, assess equipment repair needs and take corrective action
- Setting up a team "huddle" at the start of each shift to pass on each patient's requirements for toileting, transferring, and repositioning
- Providing inservice demonstrations on correct use of equipment

As the largest segment of the healthcare workforce, nurses have a powerful voice. Collectively, we must lead the transformation of the nursing work environment to preserve the viability of our profession and to keep patients safe.

CASE STUDY: IMPLEMENTATION OF A TRANSFER TEAM

Linda R. is a senior staff nurse on a long-term care unit specializing in the care of patients with Alzheimer's disease. Recently, Linda noticed that an increasing number of co-workers were complaining of back and neck strain related to transferring residents out of bed. She also observed that residents were not being turned and repositioned in bed as often as necessary. Despite an ample supply of mechanical lifting devices on the unit, Linda noted that during peak work periods, some staff members did not consistently use the mechanical lifts because they felt rushed during patient care.

Unfreezing—Clarifying the Problem

Linda approached her nurse manager with concerns about the risk of injury to staff and residents during patient transfers. Her nurse manager was in agreement, and shared that she had been alarmed by the increase in staff injuries. Additionally, the nurse manager had recently received multiple complaints from family members of residents related to their observation that residents were not being turned and repositioned often enough. She invited Linda to do a library search to explore best practices in safe patient handling and movement.

After reviewing a number of current articles, Linda identified the concept of a lift and turn team as an intervention with potential for successful implementation on her unit. Linda presented this idea of a resident transfer team to her nurse manager, explaining that a dedicated team could accomplish nearly all of the patient lifts, transports, and turns to free up nurses for other patient care responsibilities. The nurse manager agreed that Linda's proposal held promise, but advised her that this type of intervention would need to be accomplished using existing staffing resources. From the literature, Linda learned that a successful lift team could consist of a two to four specially trained nursing assistants assigned on the day shift, when the majority of patient transfers occurred.

It was important to assess staff and resident perceptions about a transfer team. Before presenting the concept of a transfer team to staff and residents, Linda recognized that she needed to assess factors in the current situation on her unit that would support implementation of a lift team (driving forces) as well as potential barriers or obstacles (restraining forces).

Linda obtained the number of nursing injuries over the past year from her nurse manager. There was clear evidence that nursing back injuries were on the rise. Several new staff members had openly admitted that they were not comfortable using the mechanical lifting devices on the unit because they had not received sufficient training. These factors were driving forces that supported the implementation of a resident transfer team. The nurse manager's commitment to improving staff and patient safety was also a driving force.

On the other hand, the fact that the transfer team had to be acquired from existing staffing was a considerable barrier or restraining force. Could any of the current-nursing assistants be persuaded to serve on the transfer team? Linda's nurse manager suggested that they partner with the other long-term care unit to see if that unit's manager and staff would be interested in pooling resources to create a transfer team comprising four nursing assistants. This team would also assume responsibility for transporting residents to appointments off the unit.

The nurse manager suggested to Linda that providing a certified, 2-day training program and a cash monetary award would offer an incentive to nursing assistants to apply for the team. The nursing assistants on the long-term care units were highly skilled in performing a variety of patient care tasks—How would other staff members perceive donating two nursing assistant positions from each unit to create a resident transfer team?

Linda enlisted Carlos, a respected nursing peer from the other long-term care unit to collect data in support of a resident transfer team. The nurse managers provided Linda and Carlos with the number of nursing injuries related to patient handling for the past year, so that they could include this information in a presentation to the staff. Linda and Carlos initiated logs to collect data over a 1-week period to show the volume of lifts and transfers on their units, as further supporting justification for a transfer team.

After collecting this information, Linda and Carlos met the nurses on their units to describe the concept of a resident transfer team and to share results of the impact of a lift team on reducing nursing back injuries. They explained that lift teams were studied in 10 hospitals and reduced injury rates by almost 70% (Charney, 2003). They included the prospect that a transfer team of four highly trained nursing assistants would free nurses from up to 95% of patient lifts, turns, and transports, so that nurses could concentrate on other direct care responsibilities. Transfer team members would always be paired up to use mechanical devices for safe performance of resident transfers and turns. The staff gave their consensus approval for implementation of a lift and turn team.

To appeal to the family members of residents, Linda and Carlos attended the resident's family support group to describe the benefits of a transfer team and solicit their support to this patient safety intervention. Family members agreed that a dedicated lift and turn team would be a positive change. Linda, Carlos, and their nurse managers met with the Nurse Executive to also acquire her support for their safe patient handling intervention project. The nurse managers obtained administrative approval from the Nurse Executive for the lift and turn team to receive a $1000 cash award per person upon completion of an intensive training program.

Moving to a New Level

Nursing staff and physical therapists were involved in developing an administrative policy for the transfer team and planning the educational program to train the team. Staff members participated as instructors in the educational program.

Additionally, staff nurses were involved in interviewing and selecting the resident transfer team. Selection criteria for the transfer team included dependable work attendance, able to meet the physical demands of the position, and excellent communication skills. Staff determined the hours of duty for the lift and turn team, based on peak workload for these activities. They decided that transfer team members would carry cell phones to facilitate access to them. Staff nurses also contributed to development of a specific job description for the transfer team.

Interdisciplinary colleagues on the long-term care units and staff from other departments were informed of the availability of the new resident transfer team, through e-mail correspondence, promotional flyers, and inservice education.

Refreezing

To assess the success of the resident transfer team, Linda and Carlos developed an evaluation plan in collaboration with their nurse managers.

They set the goal that the transfer team would absorb 95% of all resident lifts and transfers. Additionally, they identified specific outcome measures to monitor over time, including the volume of lifts, turns, and transports performed by the team, nursing injuries and lost work days, and resident/family and staff satisfaction with the transfer team. Surveys and focus groups were used to collect information about staff and resident/family satisfaction with the transfer team. Additionally, transfer team members were asked to rate their satisfaction with their roles and share issues and suggestions for improvement.

Linda and Carlos served as team leaders for the transfer team, acting as primary contacts for issues that arose during initial stages of implementation. Their continued assistance and support helped to facilitate open communication and active problem solving between the transfer team and other members of the nursing staff. The nurse manager discussed the progress and outcomes of the transfer team in monthly staff meetings to show her continued support and facilitate a smooth implementation. Over time, the resident transfer team became an integral part of the unit's safety program. Linda and Carlos presented this successful planned change and ergonomic intervention as a poster during the organization's accreditation Joint Commission (JCAHO) site visit. To their delight, the resident transfer team was recognized by JCAHO surveyors as an exemplary quality improvement.

REFERENCES

American Nurses Association Position Statement (June 21, 2003). Elimination of Manual Patient Handling to Prevent Work-Related Musculoskeletal Disorders. Retrieved April 1, 2005, from http://www.ana.org

American Nurses Association Press Release (September 17, 2003). ANA Launches 'Handle with Care' Ergonomics Campaign. Retrieved April 1, 2005, from http://www.nursingworld.org/handlewithcare

Charney, W. (1997). The lift team method for reducing back injuries: a 10 hospital study. *AAOHN Journal, 6*(45), 300–304.

Dixon, N. (2000). Common knowledge: How companies thrive by sharing what they know. Boston: Harvard Business School Press.

de Castro, A. B. (2004). Handle with care: The American Nurses Association's campaign to address work-related musculoskeletal disorders. *Online Journal of Issues in Nursing, September 30, 2004.* Retrieved April 15, 2005, from http://nursingworld.org/ojin/topic25/tpc25_2.htm

Institute of Medicine (2001). *Crossing the quality chasm: A new health system for the 21st century. Committee on the Quality of Health Care in America: Board on Health Care Services.* Washington, D.C.: National Academy Press.

Institute of Medicine (2004). Keeping patients safe: Transforming the work environment of nurses. In A. Page (Ed.), *Committee on the work environment for nurses and patient safety: Board on Health Care Services*. Washington, D.C.: National Academy Press.

Kotler, P., Roberto, N., & Lee, N. (2002). *Social marketing: Improving the quality of life* (2nd ed.). Thousand Oaks, CA: Sage Publications, Inc.

Lewin, K. (1947). Frontiers in group dynamics. *Human Relations*, (1)26–41.

Matz, M. (2006). New education model: Unit-based peer leaders. In A. Nelson (Ed.), *Handle with care: A practice guide for safe patient handling & movement* (Chap. 9). New York, NY: Springer Publishing.

Matz, M. (2006). After-action reviews. In A. Nelson (Ed.), *Handle with care: A practice guide for safe patient handling & movement* (Chap. 7). New York, NY: Springer Publishing.

Nelson, A. (October 2001 [rev. April 2005]). *Patient care ergonomics resource guide: Safe patient handling and movement*. Tampa, Florida: Patient Safety Center of Inquiry, Veterans Health Administration and Department of Defense. Purser, R., & Petranker, J. (2004). Unfreezing the future: exploring the dynamic of time in organizational change. *The Journal of Applied and Behavioral Science, 10*(20), 1–22.

Smith, N. (1996). Progression towards a 'no manual lifting' policy within the intensive care unit. *Nursing in Critical Care, 5*(1), 237–240.

Wheelan, S., Pepitone, E., & Abt, V. (Eds.). (1990). *Advances in field theory*. Newbury Park, CA: Sage Publications, Inc.

Appendix:

Sample Safe Lifting Policy for Hospitals/Nursing Homes

PURPOSE AND SCOPE OF THE POLICY

(Facility name) safe patient/resident lifting policy is one part of a comprehensive program to prevent musculoskeletal injuries to frontline caregivers, one of our most valuable resources. The policy recommends guidelines to ensure that the transferring needs of all patients/residents[1] are assessed. All healthcare personnel responsible for transferring patients shall be aware and trained on the correct procedures for lifting and moving patients. Adherence to this policy ensures that patients/residents are being lifted and transferred safely while encouraging patient mobility and independence.

Staff Responsibilities

The *Administrator* is responsible for:

1. Supporting the implementation of this policy.
2. Providing training opportunities for all staff affected by the safe-lifting policy.

---

[1]The appropriate term should be used by the health care facility; "patient" is used in hospitals, "client" in home care, and the term "resident" should be used in nursing homes.

3. Furnishing sufficient lifting equipment and repositioning aids.
4. Identifying acceptable storage locations for lifting equipment/ aids.
5. Providing resources needed for the medical management program and the evaluation of the safe-lifting program.

The unit/nurse manager, the physical and occupational therapy departments, and frontline caregivers are responsible for:

1. Assessing the transferring needs of each patient and prescribing lifting and transferring method(s) that are consistent with the patient's care plan and rehabilitation goals, ability to ambulate, bear weight, and follow verbal instructions. Patients should be reassessed if their condition changes.

Unit/nurse manager and supervisors are responsible for:

1. Ensuring that all staff affected by the policy complete initial and annual training.
2. Ensuring that the transferring needs of patients are assessed and all high-risk patient handling tasks are completed safely using mechanical lifting devices or other appropriate equipment or techniques.
3. Ensuring that mechanical lifting devices, slings, and other equipment are available, maintained in proper working order, and stored conveniently and safely.
4. Ensuring that patient transfers are being performed as prescribed.
5. Maintaining training records.

Nursing staff and frontline caregivers are responsible for:

1. Being knowledgeable of the procedures to follow when transferring patients.
2. Using proper techniques, mechanical lifting devices, and other approved equipment/aids when performing high-risk patient handling tasks.
3. Notifying supervisor if a change has occurred in a patient's condition.
4. Notifying supervisor if you have a need for retraining in the use of mechanical lifting devices, other equipment/aids, and lifting/ moving techniques.
5. Notifying supervisor if mechanical devices, slings, or equipment/ aids are damaged or need repair.
6. Notifying supervisor of any injury sustained to staff or patients.

Maintenance personnel are responsible for:

1. Inspecting the patient lifting equipment, slings, and batteries each month.
2. Maintaining lifting devices and other equipment in good working order.
3. Establishing procedures for removing damaged equipment from service.

Patient Assessment

The transferring needs of each patient should be assessed and the most appropriate lifting and transferring method(s) should be prescribed based on the patient's rehabilitation goals, ability to ambulate, bear-weight, and follow verbal instructions. Patient algorithms should be used to assess a patient's transferring needs and to identify the most appropriate methods to lift and move the patient.

Workplace Assessment

The patient care environment should be assessed to examine the layout of patient care rooms, bathrooms, and bathing areas to identify factors that might contribute to patient handling incidents, such as furniture that might interfere with transfers, the adjustability of bed height, the size of the bathrooms and bathing areas and physical barriers such as thresholds that are not level with the floor that might restrict the movement of lifting equipment.

Training Requirements

Training should be provided to all staff affected by the safe patient lifting program; this should include administrators, nursing staff, physical and occupational therapists, maintenance staff, and housekeeping and laundry staff. All nursing staff and caregivers who lift and transfer patients should be trained and made competent in the use of patient lifting equipment and procedures to follow while transferring patients. Training should be provided during employee orientation, and whenever there is a change in job assignment, equipment, or procedures. Refresher training should be conducted annually and upon the request of staff.

Equipment Requirements

The employer will provide mechanical patient lifts, slings, batteries, and repositioning aids that are made of durable quality and intended for commercial use. The number of lifts required to ensure the safety of patients and caregivers depends on the level of physical dependency of the patients. As a general rule, one full-body lift should be provided for every 8–10 non-weight bearing patients/residents, and one stand-up lift should be provided for every 8–10 partially weight-bearing residents.

Infection Control Considerations

All patient lifting equipment, slings, and assistive devices should be cleaned and laundered to comply with infection control procedures and policies. If possible, disposable slings should be used on patients who pose an infection control risk. If reusable slings are used, the patients' name should be marked on the sling and the sling should be stored at their bedside. Patient lifting equipment should be cleaned on a regular basis and after each use with a patient who poses an infection control risk.

Full-body lifts are intended for patients that cannot bear weight during any patient transferring task. If any caregiver is required to lift more than 35 lbs. of a patient's weight or the patient is unpredictable or prone to lose balance, that patient should be considered fully dependent and assistive devices should be used for the transfer. Full-body lifts can be equipped with a weighing scale.

Full-body lifts:

- Should be able to lift patients from bed height as well as pick a patient up from the floor
- Should be stored with slings in a convenient location
- Batteries should be charged when the lift is not in use

Stand-assist lifts are intended for patients with partial weight-bearing ability that require the caregiver to lift no more than 35 lbs. of a patient's weight. The patient should require no more help than stand-by, cueing, or coaxing, and the patient should have the mental capacity to follow simple commands when prompted. The stand-up lift is useful for toileting residents and for bed to chair transfers.

Stand-assist lifts:

- Should be stored in a convenient location with slings
- Batteries should be charged when the lift is not in use

Slings that are used with mechanical lifts:

- Should be available in a range of sizes
- Should be stored in a convenient location that is readily accessible to caregivers

- Back-up slings should be available for use when slings are being laundered
- Should be washable or disposable
- Should be laundered on site if possible; laundering off site can result in lost slings

Repositioning aids should be available to assist with repositioning patients/residents in bed.

Surface friction-reducing devices, slide sheets, and lateral transferring devices:

- Should be made of durable quality
- Should be capable of adjusting patients/residents in bed, regardless of patient size

Medical Management Program

If an employee is injured on the job, employees should report the injury to their supervisor immediately. Every injury should be treated promptly and each incident should be investigated so that preventive measures can be implemented.

Record Keeping

Training records shall be maintained by the training coordinator. All injury and illness records and incident investigations should be maintained and periodically examined to evaluate the effectiveness of the safe patient lifting program. Periodic analysis of these data will make it possible to identify and understand persistent injury problems and propose countermeasures.

Glossary

Administrative Controls   Procedures and methods, set up by the employer, that significantly reduce exposure to risk factors by altering the way in which work is performed. Examples include employee rotation, job task enlargement, and adjustment of work pace.

After-Action Review (AAR)   AAR is a method for transferring knowledge that a team has learned from doing a task in one setting, to the next time the same task is performed in a different setting.

Air-Assisted Lateral Transfer System   A specialty transfer mattress is installed beneath a dependent patient, onto which a portable air supply is attached that inflates the mattress. Air flows through perforations in the underside of the mattress, reducing the forces required to execute a lateral transfer.

Algorithm   A step-by-step problem-solving procedure, especially an established, recursive computational procedure for solving a problem in a finite number of steps.

Ambulation   To walk from place to place; move about.

Assistive Devices   Devices used to facilitate safe patient handling and movement.

Awkward Posture   Awkward positioning of the body while performing work activities, which may increase risk for injury. It is generally considered that the more a joint deviates from the neutral (natural) position, the greater is the risk of injury.

Back Belt   Originally made of leather, back belts are now usually made of lightweight, breathable synthetic material, and have at least one strap that tightens or loosens them.

Back Injury Resource Nurse (BIRN)   A term used within the VA to identify the unit-based Peer Safety Leader (see below).

Bariatrics   The branch of medicine that deals with the causes, prevention, and treatment of obesity.

247

Barrier Free Barrier-free building consists of building or facilities that can be used by the physically disadvantaged or disabled.

Biomechanical Loading The effects of internal and external forces on the human body.

Biomechanics Biomechanics is the field of study, which applies the laws of physics and engineering concepts to describe motion of body segments, and the forces which act upon them during activity.

Body Mass Index (BMI) The BMI can be calculated by dividing the patient's weight (in kg) by the patient's height squared (in m^2).

Body Mechanics A system for positioning the caregiver's body during patient handling and movement; once thought to protect from musculoskeletal risk but not supported by evidence.

Ceiling-Mounted Patient Lifts Ceiling-mounted patient lifts can be used safely for patients who are at times combative, unpredictable, or have cognitive deficits. These lifting devices can be used for almost any type of lift transfer.

Change Agent Those that use a systematic planning process to gain support for new ideas, procedures, and technology.

Cognition The mental process of knowing, including aspects such as awareness, perception, reasoning, and judgment.

Combative Eager or disposed to fight; belligerent.

Contracture An abnormal, often permanent shortening, as of muscle or scar tissue, that results in distortion or deformity, especially of a joint of the body.

Cost–Benefit Analysis A method of reaching economic decisions by comparing the costs of doing something with its benefits.

Demographics The characteristics of human populations and population segments.

Design A preliminary sketch or outline showing the main features of something to be executed.

Engineering Control Physical changes to jobs that control exposure to risk. Engineering controls act on the source of the hazard and control employee exposure to the hazard without relying on the employee to take self-protective action or intervention. Examples include: changing the handle angle of a tool, using a lighter weight part, and providing a chair that has adjustability.

Epidemiology The branch of medicine that deals with the study of the causes, distribution, and control of disease in populations.

Ergonomics The scientific study of the relation between people and their occupation, equipment and environment. In simple terms, ergonomics is designing for human use.

Etiology   A branch of knowledge concerned with causes, specifically a branch of medical science concerned with the causes and origins of diseases.

Friction-Reducing Devices   Often constructed of smooth synthetic fabrics, these devices offer friction-reducing properties to facilitate the lateral transfer or repositioning of patients that can offer limited or no assistance. They effectively reduce the forces required to execute the transfer, minimizing biomechanical loading on the caregiver's arms and back. Properly designed handles and pull straps can improve the caregivers' grasp and reduce forward reach during transfers.

Gait/Transfer Belt   An object with handles is often easier to grasp. Patients wear this belt, with convenient handles for the caregiver(s) to grasp when assisting the transfer of a partially dependent patient.

Injury Incidence Rate (IIR)   Total number of injuries/hours worked by all employees $\times$ 200,000 = IIR.

Institute of Medicine   In the United States, the Institute of Medicine serves as adviser to the nation to improve health. As an independent, scientific adviser, the Institute of Medicine strives to provide advice that is unbiased, based on evidence, and grounded in science.

Knowledge Management   The goal of knowledge management is to ensure needed knowledge is made available by fostering the sharing of information.

Knowledge Transfer   For the purposes of this book, this is the transmission of information intended to effect actions taken in response to hazardous conditions/circumstances in the healthcare work environment, thus decreasing risk of injury.

Lateral Transfer   Lateral transfers (patient starts and ends lying in a prone or supine position), such as bed to stretcher, bed to prone cart, or bed to bath trolley.

Lift Team   Two or more patient caregivers organized in a team with primary responsibility of performing patient lifts and transfers within a healthcare facility, using appropriate equipment and techniques. Lift team members receive specialized training to ensure their competence in the performance of a variety of high-risk patient lifts and transfers.

Loading   The pressure on the spine.

Macroscopic   Considered in terms of large units or elements in a system.

Mechanical Lateral Transfer Aids   Those devices that provide mechanized or powered assistance for patient horizontal transfers and therefore eliminate the need to manually slide patients, substantially reducing the risk of injury to caregivers.

Medicaid   In the United States, a joint federal and state program that helps with medical costs for some people with low incomes and limited resources. Medicaid programs vary from state to state, but most health care costs are covered if you qualify for both Medicare (see below) and Medicaid.

Medicare   In the United States, the federal health insurance program for people 65 years of age or older, certain younger people with disabilities, and people with End-Stage Renal Disease (permanent kidney failure with dialysis or a transplant, sometimes called ESRD).

Mesoscopic   Considered in terms of middle range units or elements in a system.

Microscopic   Considered in terms of small units or elements in a system.

Mobility   The quality or state of being able to move readily from place to place.

Mock-Up   A full-sized structural model built accurately to scale chiefly for study, testing, or display.

Musculoskeletal Disorders   Injuries and disorders of the muscles, nerves, tendons, ligaments, joints, cartilage, and spinal disc. Examples include carpal tunnel syndrome, rotator cuff tendonitis, and epicondylitis.

National Institute for Occupational Safety and Health (NIOSH)   Federal government agency under the United States Department of Health and Human Services established to help assure safe and healthful working conditions for working men and women by providing research, information, education, and training in the field of occupational safety and health.

Occupational Illness   Any abnormal condition or disorder, other than one resulting from an occupational injury caused by exposure to factors associated with employment. It includes acute and chronic illnesses or disease, which may be caused by inhalation, absorption, ingestion, or direct contact. The broad categories of occupational illnesses are skin diseases and disorders, dust diseases of the lungs, respiratory condition due to toxic agents, poisoning (systemic effects of toxic materials), disorders due to physical agents other than toxic materials, and disorders from repeated trauma.

Occupational Injuries   Any injury such as a cut, fracture, sprain, amputation, etc., which results from a work-related event or from a single instantaneous exposure in the work environment.

Occupational Safety and Health Administration (OSHA)   Government agency under the United States Department of Labor with the mission to assure the safety and health of America's workers by setting and enforcing standards; providing training, outreach, and education; establishing partnerships; and encouraging continual improvement in workplace safety and health.

OSHA 300 Log   An OSHA-required (see above) form for employers to record and classify occupational injuries and illnesses, and note the extent of each case.

Patient Lifting Equipment Category of equipment that lift patients either in a seated or supine position from one place to another. This category includes ceiling lifts, floor-based lifts, and sit-to-stand lifts.

Peer Safety Leaders (Unit-Based) Implement and maintain patient care ergonomic program elements, facilitate knowledge transfer on program elements and equipment, act as unit experts and resources on patient care ergonomics and equipment, champion the patient care ergonomic cause, and monitor and evaluate the program.

Powered Positioning Allows the caregiver the facility to change a patient's posture using the powered advantage of the patient lift system. This new technology is available for both floor-based and ceiling-mounted patient lifts.

Powered Transport Devices These devices can be attached to the head of bed or stretcher and are motorized to assist in propulsion of the patient. This low-cost device can be used for patient transport throughout a hospital or nursing home, requiring only one caregiver to perform the task. Some newer higher end stretchers and hospital beds have integrated motorized capability.

Qualitative Information The separation of an intellectual or material whole into its constituent parts (the nature of the material) for individual study, including the study of such constituent parts and their interrelationships in making up a whole (as opposed to quantitative analysis, or the separation of elements to determine their proportion).

Repetitive Motion Injuries Damage to tendons, nerves, and other soft tissues, which is caused by the repeated performance of a limited number of physical movements and is characterized by numbness, pain, and muscles weakness.

Repositioning Adjusting patient's position in a bed or chair to prevent pressure ulcers and promote comfort.

Risk Factor Actions in the workplace, workplace conditions, or a combination thereof, which may cause or aggravate work-related musculoskeletal disorders. Examples include forceful exertion, awkward postures, repetitive exertion, and environmental factors such as temperature.

Safe Lifting Policy One part of a comprehensive approach to preventing musculoskeletal injuries to health care workers. The intent of the policy should be to establish the minimum standards for safe patient lifting by providing written guidelines that can be used by health care administrators, supervisors, and frontline employees to allocate resources and understand and apply the elements of a safe patient handling and movement program. The basic premise that manual handling of patients should be avoided where possible (also referred to as "zero-lift," "minimal lift," or "no-manual-lift," or "no-lift policy").

Simulation   The imitative representation of the functioning of one system or process by means of the functioning of another.

Social Marketing   A process designed to sell ideas to influence a target audience to change behavior.

Supine   Lying on the back or having the face upward.

Task Analysis   Provide an assessment of the caregiver's exposure to physical risk factors that can contribute to musculoskeletal disorders.

Torque   A force that produces or tends to produce rotation or torsion; also a measure of the effectiveness of such a force that consists of the product of the force and the perpendicular distance from the line of action of the force to the axis of rotation; a turning or twisting force.

Transfer Chairs   Some new wheelchairs and dependency chairs can convert into stretchers where the back of the chair pulls down and the leg supports come up to form a flat stretcher. These devices facilitate the horizontal transfer of patients between the chair and bed or stretcher, thereby eliminating the need to perform a vertical transfer.

US Bureau of Labor Statistics (BLS)   United States governmental agency providing safety and health statistics concerning occupational injuries and illnesses. Generally regarded as reliable by the industry.

US Department of Labor   United States governmental agency charged with issues relating to workplace safety and health, pensions and benefit plans, employment, and other issues related to the American workplace.

Vertical Transfer   Patient starts and ends in a seated position, such as transfer from bed to chair, chair to toilet, wheelchair to bedside chair, or car to wheelchair.

Veterans Health Administration (VHA)   Provides a broad spectrum of medical, surgical, and rehabilitative care to veterans.

Work-Related Musculoskeletal Disorders (WMSD, WRMSD)   Injuries and disorders of the muscles, nerves, tendons, ligaments, joints, cartilage, and spinal disc due to physical work activities or workplace conditions in the job. Examples include carpal tunnel syndrome, rotator cuff tendonitis, and epicondylitis.

Workload   The amount of work assigned to or expected from a worker in a specified time period.

Index

Page numbers followed by f or t indicate figures or tables, respectively.